Public Health, Mental Health and Human Rights

Public Health, Mental Health and Human Rights:

The Example of North Iraq

Edited by

Jan Ilhan Kizilhan, Anna Weigelt, Julia Beckmann and Thomas Wenzel

Cambridge Scholars
Publishing

Public Health, Mental Health and Human Rights:
The Example of North Iraq

Edited by Jan Ilhan Kizilhan, Anna Weigelt, Julia Beckmann and Thomas Wenzel

This book first published 2025

Cambridge Scholars Publishing

Lady Stephenson Library, Newcastle upon Tyne, NE6 2PA, UK

British Library Cataloguing in Publication Data
A catalogue record for this book is available from the British Library

ISBN: 978-1-0364-4911-7
ISBN (Ebook): 978-1-0364-4912-4

TABLE OF CONTENTS

PREFACE I

THERESIA BAUER

MEMBER OF THE STATE PARLIAMENT
OF BADEN-WÜRTTEMBERG, GERMANY

When thousands of refugees came from Iraq to the state of Baden-Württemberg in Germany in 2015 and 2016, we knew immediately that we had to do more than make offers for integration in our country. It seemed just as important to us to initiate projects in the regions affected, to address, or at least mitigate, their causes of flight.

For example, the Kurdistan Region of Iraq, which has more than five million inhabitants, has taken in more than two million internally displaced persons and refugees. This is an enormous challenge for the region and we wanted to provide targeted assistance here. As early as 2015, the state of Baden-Württemberg therefore established a collaborative agreement with the Duhok governorate, which was extended in 2019 during a delegation trip with the former Minister of State, Theresa Schopper, and myself.

Examples of aid initiatives on the ground were a carpet manufactory in Khanke, in which women affected by war and displacement could build their own livelihood, and the construction of a regenerative power supply in the Mam Rashan refugee camp. However, the centerpiece of our relief efforts was a Special Quota Project in which particularly vulnerable women and their children were relocated from northern Iraq to Baden-Württemberg. In 2015 and 2016, we took in around 1,100 particularly vulnerable women and children from Iraq, many of them of the Yazidi faith. These were women who had been held captive and tortured by the terrorist organization Islamic State. They received psychotherapeutic help in Baden-Württemberg and were supported on their way back to a safe life.

As a logical next step, especially following our experiences with the Special Quota Project, an idea developed in late fall 2016 to establish an Institute for Psychotherapy and Psychotraumatology at the University of Duhok, and to set-up a master's degree program in psychotraumatology. I was particularly convinced by the fact that expertise would be built up locally in northern Iraq to help people there right from the start of the project.

After the urgent need for such an institute was recognized by all sides, everyone involved worked intensively on the design of the institute. After initial drafts in the fall of 2016, a final application was submitted by the Dual University of Baden-Württemberg (DHBW) at the beginning of 2017. It was immediately reviewed and approved by the Ministry of Science. The Institute for Psychotherapy and Psychotraumatology at the University of Duhok was then launched in March 2017.

There is no blueprint for such a project, but the Ministry has recognized expertise in the support and establishment of institutes and study programs in Baden-Württemberg. As such, we were able to build on this knowledge. The project leaders, Professor Kizilhan from the Baden-Württemberg Cooperative State University and Professor Hautzinger from the University of Tübingen, are two distinguished, internationally experienced, and recognized academics who are held in high esteem locally in northern Iraq. The project was also supported by the former governor of Duhok. The administration of the University of Duhok was very committed to the project and took care of the constructional requirements.

Of course, there were challenges in transferring funds from Baden-Württemberg to northern Iraq, with evidence and documentation required under our budgetary law. A very precise documentation and description of the administrative processes was absolutely necessary. When problems arose, the project participants, their budget departments at the universities, and representatives from my office sat down together and worked out solutions. When visas were needed for lecturers from Baden-Württemberg, we supported the visa application process with accompanying letters. In addition, the university administration from Duhok visited us regularly in Stuttgart to report on project progress and problems. During a delegation trip to Duhok in April 2019, we were also able to see the progress of the project, the work in the refugee camps, and the high motivation of the students. Directly experiencing tense situations on the ground, and having conversations with refugees in the camps, showed us how important and correct the decision was to support the project.

The project has achieved more than laying a foundation for care and therapy in a crisis area; it has also broken down cultural skepticism about psychotherapy locally. The people there have learned that altruistic help is available, especially for women and children, who are among the most vulnerable victims of war. We have spoken with local dignitaries and responsible ministers to ensure continuation of the work on site.

During the project, we also had to accept that the project might be interrupted due to war-related interventions. Indeed, in 2018, flights to Erbil were no longer possible because the airport was closed for a short time. Support and teaching then continued digitally. The project with the university and the region of Duhok is not comparable with other projects in Baden-Württemberg. It is a project in a crisis region where people have had to endure existential challenges for years. In addition, the geographical proximity to Islamic State (IS) territory must not be forgotten. Just 70 kilometers from Duhok lies Mosul, a former stronghold of the IS. We would read daily newspapers quite differently and fervently hoped that no project partners were endangered. The "safety first" message was always important and the health of those involved in the project was of great concern to us in Baden-Württemberg.

I hope that the project will inspire many imitators. Every day the news shows more than 80 million people are on the run and suffer harm to body and soul. If we are able to make a significant contribution to solving this problem, I would be very happy. I am very grateful that I was able to support this project and visit it on site.

PREFACE II

PROF. DR. DAWOOD SULEIMAN ATRUSHI

PRESIDENT OF THE UNIVERSITY OF DUHOK

In the aftermath of the Islamic State of Iraq and Syria (ISIS) invasion of the Kurdistan Region of Iraq, with all the tragedies and atrocities they caused to different civilian communities, a huge number of people needed urgent health care support, including mental health care services. Due to years of war and conflict in the region, the health care system had become compromised and there was a lack of mental health professionals to meet the needs of the affected communities. Thankfully, Professor Ilhan Kizilhan had a comprehensive understanding of the context at the time and sought to find a solution or establish an institution in coordination with the University of Duhok to tackle these critical challenges and mental health needs of our region.

Professor Kizilhan played a key role in making a connection between the University of Duhok and the Ministry of Science and Culture in Baden-Württemberg in Germany, to support a project that would have sustainable impact locally, while educating and training mental health professionals in the region. Consequently, the decision to establish the Institute for Psychotherapy and Psychotraumatology (IPP) was made.

This was a great step towards achieving the overall objective of supporting the mental health system in the region, especially in response to the trauma and the tragedies inflicted by ISIS. As the president of the University of Duhok, I appreciated the efforts that Professor Ilhan Kizilhan put into this idea and the project, due to its significant importance. That is why I have decided to make sure that all the support needed by the University of Duhok is provided, to facilitate the implementation of the project here as much as possible.

Before starting the project, we had many meetings with the professors and faculty members from the University of Tübingen, to conduct needs assessments for the requirements of this joint project. The discussion focused on provision of a curriculum that considered a variety of academic aspects from both Germany and the Kurdistan region. The core scientific curriculum of an academic field is almost the same anywhere in the world, but the delivery can sometimes differ from one country to another. However, we at the University of Duhok are very open to incorporate new teaching and learning methods into our system. We believe that the IPP has succeeded in offering learning and training methods in psychology and psychotraumatology, and we appreciate that.

Therefore, I think that the IPP is a good example of international collaboration in scientific and education fields. A project like this does not only respond to the critical needs of psychology and psychotraumatology. This project may create opportunities for mutual understanding and learning between communities. We at the University of Duhok are thinking about establishing a new project with the German University. For example, we are thinking of establishing a joint B.Sc. degree in Psychology between our university and one of the German universities.

Furthermore, I believe that the IPP is a true example of sustainable development. The project will have a long lasting and community-wide effect for decades to come. Graduates of this institution are local, and will be entering the local system, which will benefit from the knowledge and skills that they have gained during their studies. I believe that the growing need for mental health support and services in this region will be the biggest factor in preserving the IPP in the future.

Before, in the Kurdistan region, patients with psychological problems had to be sent to Europe or outside Kurdistan to get treatment, and they had the problem of applying for a visa. Some of them were asking for refugee status or political asylum, creating problems with organizations abroad. But now we have our own specialists who can treat these people without needing to go abroad.

Having said that, I would like to thank Professor Ilhan Kizilhan, the Institute for Transcultural Health Science, and its associates and network for their efforts and help. Finally, I would like to express my sincere thanks to the Ministry of Science and Culture at State of Baden-Württemberg, the Foreign Ministry in Germany, and the German Academic Exchange Service (DAAD) for their continuous help and support to our university and region in general.

PREFACE III

PROF. DR. MARTIN HAUTZINGER

UNIVERSITY OF TÜBINGEN

What a strange idea: We need more engineers, physicians, soldiers, and administrators, but no psychotherapists. Wrong!

Nobody denies that we need all of these professions, but a large part of the population suffers from psychological problems and need help. In post-war regions, especially in low-income countries, a health care system does not exist, is far from qualified, and requires support. They need psychological experts and psychotherapists to overcome trauma and heal psychological wounds. For example, after the terror of ISIS in 2014 and the war in Syria, many people took refuge in the Kurdistan Region of Iraq (KRI). Many governmental projects and non-Government organizations (NGOs) that work in this region have focused on giving shelter (tents), organizing basic medical services and childcare, and providing short term advice and counseling. But a large proportion of refugees and tortured people suffer with severe mental illness, in particular posttraumatic stress disorder (PTSD) and depression. First line, evidence-based treatment for these disorders is psychotherapy (Cognitive Behavior Therapy (CBT) according to the well-established independent UK National Institute for Clinical Excellence (NICE) guidelines), which is not available in this region.

With our expertise in CBT, and PTSD, implementing training, supervising therapists, and teaching on different academic levels, we convinced our state and federal government, as well as private sponsors, to support the development of an academic program in Kurdistan. It was the University of Duhok who was open for our "educational adventure" by starting the Institute for Psychotherapy and Psychotraumatology (IPP). The IPP's 3-year master's program teaches students who already have a bachelor's degree either in Psychology or Social Work to become professional psychotherapists, with theoretical, diagnostic, and therapeutic competence to treat a wide variety of mental disorders. It was, and still is, our plan to establish sustainable structures for psychotherapy education as well as psychological treatment in the area.

From the beginning, we followed several principles: (a) education in evidence-based psychotherapy, (b) the training should be culture and trauma sensitive, (c) a core group of local professionals should be trained so that they can provide training for further local therapists, (d) the project should be coordinated with local leaders, the local government, health care services, and academic institutions, (e) an outpatient clinic should be established, offering psychotherapy to the public, and (f) research should be encouraged in order to educate clinicians up to doctoral level and provide more information about this region. We are convinced that real sustainability of mental health care programs can best be established by enabling local professionals to become more competent to support their communities.

Now, after almost 10 years we have reached most of these goals. We have already educated 65 psychotherapists, working in regional organizations, clinics, and administrations. They are treating patients, teaching students, and training future psychotherapists. As an extension of the IPP, we have established an outpatient clinic for psychotherapy ("German Clinic for Psychotherapy"), run by a group of our former master's students, where psychotherapy is offered for free. Currently, about 80 patients are seen and treated there. We have qualified a group of psychotherapists as instructors and supervisors to run the academic training at the IPP. A new group of students are now involved in the master's program under the instruction of the local teaching psychotherapists. After graduation, some of our former students became doctoral students, conducting research for their dissertations under our supervision.

It is a pleasure and fills me with gratitude to document our initial ideas, our goals, the (not always smooth) process to reach these goals, and where we are right now, within the chapters of this book. This documentation should help others to build up similar academic programs for the education of psychotherapists. We are convinced that instead of moving patients to countries where successful treatment is available, it is a much better option to educate local mental health workers in evidence-based psychotherapy to help their people in their country.

INTRODUCTION

JAN ILHAN KIZILHAN AND THOMAS WENZEL

In recent decades, many health care systems in high-income countries, such as Germany, Austria, the UK, and the USA, have faced increasing challenges and limitations in offering affordable health care services. This particularly affects groups of the population that depend on free health care. In recent decades, there has been a noticeable decline in the number of available healthcare experts and service providers, leading to insufficient numbers available in many regions.

Challenges in training and recruiting the necessary health care professionals have been observed, not only in the so-called "developing" countries. This has been caused by several factors, including increasing age, insufficient or unattractive working conditions, increased specialization requirements, sophistication and professionalization of the health care systems, and growing populations. The situation presents a challenging future for all health care professionals, their patients, and for public healthcare systems.

The situation is even more critical in the "developing" and low-income countries, which often suffer from a complete lack of free services, educational and training structures, more unattractive working conditions for health care professionals, and a continuous "brain drain" of the already limited number of experts. Further, these challenges are exacerbated by further difficulties in areas affected by war or civil-war, in post-conflict regions, and in larger disaster areas, such as the recent earthquake-affected regions in Turkey and Syria. During and following man-made or natural disasters, there are increased health care needs, especially for mental health care and psychological support. In some of these regions, discrimination, persecution, and even genocide affect some population groups, such as ethnic and religious minorities, more severely than others. Therefore, in addition to pre-existing problems, post-conflict and disaster regions face new problems, and groups with already insufficient access to healthcare may be at the greatest disadvantage.

This book presents the experience, evaluation and "lessons learned" from a large, long-term project that was supported by the German government and other donors and implemented in a collaboration between

German and Kurdish-Iraqi universities and their respective governments and healthcare authorities. This project aimed to address extreme mental health challenges faced in the Kurdish Region of Iraq, which was nearly devastated by war and conflict. So far, most projects addressing similar situations have been short-term, highly limited in scope, and have not focused on building long-term sustainable structures to fit existing environments, resources, and cultures in diverse affected regions.

The global increase in the already mentioned challenging healthcare situations in post-war and catastrophe countries such as Turkey, Syria, Ethiopia, Sudan, and Ukraine underline the need for evidence-based holistic approaches and models. These models should address the complex challenges faced in these catastrophic situations, which threaten whole populations, particularly minority and vulnerable groups. The authors aim therefore to use the aforementioned insights, research results, and "lessons learned" from this major project to offer guidance for the creation of sustainable interdisciplinary projects which can address the needs of populations in similarly affected countries. The book is not limited to summaries and discussions of theoretical research. Rather, alongside a synthesis of the most relevant research, concrete guidelines and sustainable solution models are presented. These have been tested in real-life environments to address public mental health problems in countries affected by conflict or other large-scale disasters.

The book consists of several sections (parts). First, a summary of the state-of-the-art knowledge on the most relevant emerging issues in the context of these challenges. This is followed by an overview of the preparatory analysis of the country and cultural background and context performed in preparation of the pilot project, which may be used as a model for further activities in Iraq and similar countries when addressing psychological health, followed by both a team-based and an external independent evaluation of the project strategy and outcomes. The authors will summarize both general and specific recommendations and tools which have resulted from the research and pilot project in detail. Relevant materials such as questionnaires, a list of team members, and other materials developed in the project are collected in the appendices at the end of the book.

We believe the materials we provide in this book can help develop similar projects and avoid pitfalls in mental health care services within these challenging environments. While the project was developed in a post-war zone, we expect that similar challenges and solutions could apply, albeit with modifications, in regions affected by large-scale natural disasters.

We are grateful for support by:

- Foreign Ministry of Germany
- Ministry for Science and Culture, State of Baden-Württemberg
- State Ministry of Baden-Württemberg
- Ministry for Higher Education, KRI
- German Academic Exchange Services (Deutscher-Akademischer Austauschdienst – DAAD)
- Ministry of Development and Cooperation
- Deutsche Gesellschaft für internationale Zusammenarbeit (GIZ)
- Eric Gustav Adler Stiftung, Germany
- Caritas International
- Schwäbische Zeitung
- Governor of Duhok
- And all network partners in Iraq, Kurdistan, Germany and worldwide

PART 1

AN OVERVIEW OF THE SCIENTIFIC DISCUSSION RELEVANT TO THE PROJECT

CHAPTER 1

MASS VIOLENCE, WAR AREAS, AND THEIR LONG-TERM MENTAL HEALTH IMPACT: FORMS OF DISCRIMINATION, GENOCIDE, AND SEVERE HUMAN RIGHTS VIOLATIONS

THOMAS WENZEL AND REEM ALKSIRI

To better understand the specific needs of different groups, we must consider the many forms of trauma experienced by survivors in diverse situations, as during mass violence, severe human rights violations, war, and civil war. Each type of violence can have different psychological, social, legal, and economic consequences. These consequences can interact in a complex way and require specific strategies to guide adequate interventions. We must also acknowledge hidden forms of violence not always immediately thought of alongside immediate physical violence. These include structural violence, different acts of discrimination, poverty, uneven distribution of resources in large population groups by political actors, the impact of environmental change, and finally, more (or less) "natural" catastrophes and their aftermath. The reaction of survivors or survivor groups might take different forms, which we will cover separately, ranging from post-traumatic growth to severe forms of complex post-traumatic stress disorder and other chronic mental health sequels. This also includes the transgenerational transmission of trauma, that, as seen in Iraq, reflect multiple historical genocides.

Genocide

Let us first look at genocide, as a traumatic event of particular relevance in Iraq. The term "genocide" was first used by the Polish-Jewish lawyer, Raphael Lemkin, in the context of what we refer to as the "Armenian genocide" today, by the Ottomans (and later "Young Turks") (Lemkin &

Bazyler, 2008). This was an event that led to the creation of the United Nations (UN) Anti-Genocide Convention (Convention on the Prevention and Punishment of the Crime of Genocide, adopted 09 December 1948, by General Assembly resolution 260 A (III), and Entry into force: 12 January 1951)[1].

The Convention defines genocide in Article II and lists events associated with it:

> "In the present Convention, genocide means any of the following acts committed with intent to destroy, in whole or in part, a national, ethnical, racial or religious group, as such:
> (a) Killing members of the group;
> (b) Causing serious bodily or mental harm to members of the group;
> (c) Deliberately inflicting on the group conditions of life calculated to bring about its physical destruction in whole or in part;
> (d) Imposing measures intended to prevent births within the group;
> (e) Forcibly transferring children of the group to another group."

It further stipulates:

> "The following acts shall be punishable:
> (a) Genocide;
> (b) Conspiracy to commit genocide;
> (c) Direct and public incitement to commit genocide;
> (d) Attempt to commit genocide;
> (e) Complicity in genocide."

This important Convention, which is clearly defined at first glance, should be upheld by the signatory countries, other countries, UN bodies, and the UN Security Council. However, as recent events have shown, effective implementation of the Convention can be hindered by political interests and legal barriers, especially relating to the interpretation of Article II. This might indicate that the broader original understanding of the definition by Lemkin should be considered and respected. Nevertheless, we do not intend to get into legal details in the context of this book.

Many groups and their advocates have been fighting for their experiences to be recognized as genocides in the UN Convention definition. This process can be long and arduous, and groups may be used as political cards in the games of political players. Examples range from Armenia, to

---

[1] See https://www.ohchr.org/en/instruments-mechanisms/instruments/convention-prevention-and-punishment-crime-genocide

the Yazidi group in northern Iraq (Kizilhan et al., 2023), the Uighurs in the Xinjiang area of China[2], the Rohingya group to ethnic groups in Dafur (Hagan & Kaiser, 2011), Indigenous people in Australia (Tatz, 2001), and US African- American and First Nations people (Tanne, 2010).

Sometimes, the response of the UN and similar global players is not immediate and efficient, or is inherently constrained by definitions and mandates. In these situations, national third-country parliaments (i.e., in the case of the Yazidi, the German Parliament) or global independent tribunals (i.e., in the Uighur case, the international tribunal[2] based in London) can take a first step to creating awareness of a problem and contributing to justice (Kizilhan & Neumann, 2020) and recognition. This is important not only for prevention, but also for the psychological recovery of the victim groups.

In the context of public health, flexible definitions might be most useful to understand the impact of genocide and, in areas like Iraq, the impact of multiple genocides. We propose the use of the term of "genocidal acts" (any activity that, if seen by itself, might be a common event but might be part of a more long-term genocidal strategy by different perpetrators) and the concept of a "genocidal environment" (i.e., a geographical or socio-political area where genocidal acts are frequent over longer periods). As we will discuss later in this chapter, medical categories and models focusing only on individuals might be insufficient to understand the psychological, biological, and social impacts of experiencing genocidal acts. This includes the development of coping strategies and (relative) resilience in some survivors, or the impacts of transgenerational trauma in other instances.

[2] See https://uyghurtribunal.com/

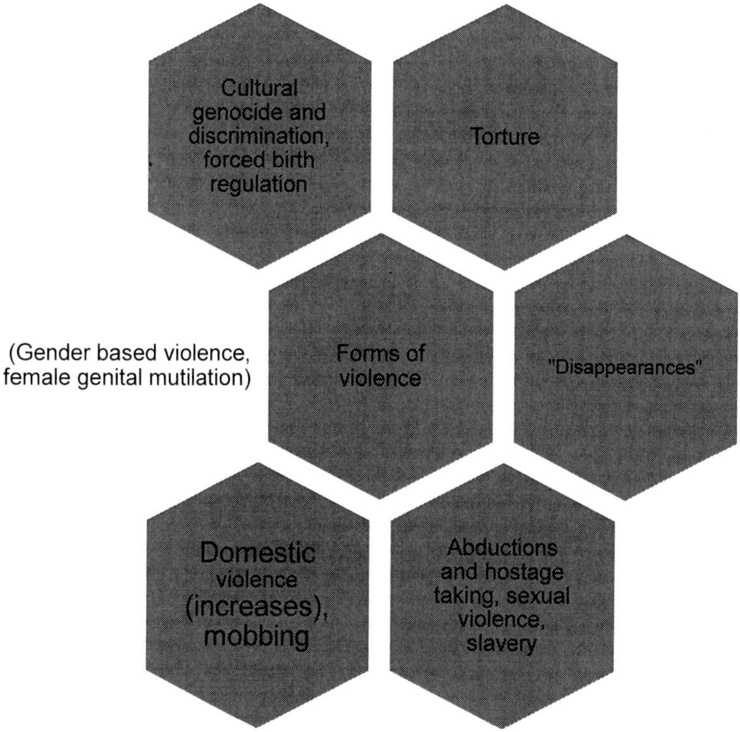

Fig. 1-1 Different forms of violence encountered (not only) in war areas and post-conflict zones

Conducting research under difficult conditions

To understand the impact of mass violence, genocidal acts, or war, we need reliable data to guide interventions and create adequate models which accurately reflect the characteristics of each situation. Science is, and probably always has been, a process that is influenced, controlled, or prohibited by political parties, despite efforts against this by the international scientific community. Efforts to ensure objective science include independent peer review, and research and publication standards. Examples include the COPE guidelines[3] on publication ethics (Committee

[3] See https://publicationethics.org/guidance/Guidelines

on Public, 2000), the World Medical Association's (WMA) Ethical guidelines[4] and specific position statements for medical research, and policies from other international professional umbrella bodies and Non-Governmental organizations (NGOs), such as the European Federation of Psychologists' Association (EFPA)[5].

In Iraq, post-conflict zones, or areas with ongoing conflict, independent research using typical methods can be difficult. However, international institutions, such as the UN or the International Criminal Court (ICC), can actively start investigating legal and other aspects of these situations. Based on their data, they can prepare legal or other interventions. They may still be hindered by challenges such as an impasse in the UN Security Council, which might inhibit their essential functions.

Research about mental health in post-conflict zones, or areas with ongoing conflict, can be especially limited when research approaches come from university settings in safe, high-income countries, without appropriate consideration of the group being studied. Factors which need to be considered include cultural aspects, differences between collective/community-oriented and individual-focused priorities in a society, the existing healthcare culture, gender influences, and prior trauma due to transgenerational transmission of the impact of earlier violence and genocidal acts, for example. Furthermore, appropriate approaches should seek to identify and include local resources for an integrated strategic approach to the research and consequent interventions

If independent legal or scientific investigations are difficult, alternative strategies have been explored to gather data on human rights abuses and their impact on a specific country. These strategies, particularly when combined in an integrative or "triangulated" manner, can provide reasonably reliable understandings of specific situations "on the ground," potentially guiding further investigations or interventions. Effective interventions might also be offered in third (host) countries, where survivors, who might be direct or indirect victims, are alive and able to escape persecution and immediate danger. This support in third countries might include different forms of redress, such as medical treatment and psychotherapy, but also other considerations, including economic support or protection like asylum status, protection against refoulement, and sometimes justice against perpetrators offered by universal jurisdiction principles (International Council on Human Rights Policy, 1999).

[4] See https://www.wma.net/what-we-do/education/medical-ethics-manual/

[5] See https://www.efpa.eu/model-code-ethics

These forms of protection and support are stipulated as obligatory in host countries by international documents such as the UN Convention against Torture and the EU reception directive[6], which defines vulnerable groups that require special consideration and support. Universal jurisdiction has recently been explored as a tool for prosecuting perpetrators in third countries if local authorities do not conduct prompt and effective investigations. However, in "transitional" justice situations, the effectiveness of this strategy might need to be considered, as it may not always offer redress to individual victims. The recent conviction of an Islamic State of Iraq and Syria (ISIS) member in a German court for crimes against a Yazidi girl, based on the principle of universal jurisdiction, highlights the potential for achieving justice in situations like those in Iraq and Syria[7].

Reliable information, independent of potentially false or biased claims in perpetrator countries, must be obtained in different ways to justify such support in third (host) countries or further interventions by international bodies. Medical and psychological examinations, following guidelines of the recently updated UN/WMA Istanbul protocol (Iacopino et al., 2022; Koseoglu, 2022), can provide objective evidence about the impacts of perpetrator actions on survivors. This evidence, combined with testimonies from witnesses and survivors may contribute to this important task. In Iraq, the Investigative Team to Promote Accountability for Crimes Committed by Da'esh/the Islamic State of Iraq and the Levant (ISIL, also known as ISIS) – UNIDAT[8]- fills this void with its independent mandate, despite facing ongoing challenges related to the extension of its authority.

Other strategies for investigation, many developed only recently, might involve the analysis of publicly available documents and sources. For example, analysis of satellite images can document mass graves or torture sites, as seen recently in Ukraine and earlier in China's Xinjiang region[9]. Pictorial evidence and other documents produced by perpetrators themselves, not initially intended for public release, can also be used. Examples of this in-

---

6 Available from
https://eur-lex.europa.eu/legal-content/EN/TXT/?uri= celex%3A32013L0033

[7] See
https://www.nytimes.com/2021/11/30/world/europe/isis-trial-yazidi-germany.html

[8] See https://www.unitad.un.org/

[9] See https://www.bbc.com/news/world-europe-61183056 and
https://www.rand.org/pubs/articles/2021/chinas-disappeared-uyghurs-what-satellite-images-reveal.html

clude the "Caesar" series in Syria[10], Nazi Germany's concentration camp-related and other relevant documents[11], published documents on torture in Argentina[12], and documents by the former regime of Iraq. These sources can be used to investigate past abuses, which can be important for several reasons: offering therapeutic justice, identifying and prosecuting perpetrators to prevent future threats, safeguarding against recurrence, defining redress - including access to free treatment for victims suffering from the consequences of human rights violations - and informing future reforms

Research in conflict zones and humanitarian disasters still needs to follow ethical standards and consider cultural differences. This issue was recently discussed by Turner and Avison (2003) who highlighted the challenge of ethics in the transcultural context across different societies. They concluded: "A more realistic recognition of multiple moral traditions in pluralist societies would be considerably more skeptic about the contributions that common morality approaches in bioethics can make to resolving contentious moral issues" (Turner & Avison, 2003).

Gender issues

Women face significant challenges due to both historical discrimination and targeted violence in conflict areas. For example, in Iraq, ISIS/DAESH targeted women with brutal violence (Kizilhan, Friedl, et al., 2020). Additionally, they face ongoing discrimination that creates barriers to reintegrating into a normal life, as outlined below.

Key guiding instruments, with a gender lens and focus on women's rights, include the Istanbul Convention[13], which addresses domestic violence, and the Bangkok Rules (UN Rules for the Treatment of Women

[10] https://www.theguardian.com/world/2015/oct/01/they-were-torturing-to-kill-inside-syrias-death-machine-caesar, accessed 5.11.2023

[11] See for example the online collection at https://www.ushmm.org/collections/plan-a-research-visit/electronic-resources/primary-source-databases, accessed 31.1.2024

[12] See https://nsarchive.gwu.edu/briefing-book/southern-cone/2020-07-21/argentinas-house-of-horrors, accessed 31.1.2024

[13] https://www.coe.int/en/web/istanbul-convention, accessed 31.1.2024, not to be confused with the Istanbul declaration on organ transplantation or the UN Istanbul Protocol for Torture related investigations

Prisoners and Non-custodial Measures for Women Offenders)[14]. Women are also becoming increasingly recognized for their important roles as human rights defenders (Correa-Chica et al., 2024; Kabengele Mpinga & Chastonay, 2005). This last development is reflected in the establishment of the International Day of Women Human Rights Defenders[15] and the creation of special institutions and programs within the UN and other organizations. Recent cases, such as the persecution and imprisonment of Prof. Sebnem Korur Fincanci, an internationally renowned forensic expert and human rights defender, highlight the risks faced by this group. Prof. Fincanci has been active in numerous, including Kurdish, areas, such as post-disaster and mass violence contexts, and has served as president of the Turkish Medical Association. Her detention sparked widespread international protests, including from the World Medical Organization (Heisler et al., 2022).

Research projects and proposed interventions must consider gender-related challenges and the needs of all genders, with a special focus on women. Gender has often been neglected in international health and medical research, as seen in examples such as differences in drug metabolism or biorhythms.

The psychosocial and legal concerns of Iraqi women were an important focus in the project presented in this book, and were addressed by gender-specific support actions. Women were not only specific targets of violence in northern Iraq (Al Shawi & Hassen, 2022), but when abducted by ISIS/DAESH terrorist groups, they faced challenges in returning to their communities (Ibrahim et al., 2018; Kizilhan, Friedl, et al., 2020; Kizilhan, Steger, et al., 2020). The traditions of their Yazidi religion prohibit "marriage" or any form of sexual contact with individuals from different groups, even if forced by terrorists like the Sunni oriented ISIS groups. Consequently, returning to their home communities after these traumatic experiences was difficult for Yazidi women, especially as former neighbors, mainly from the Sunni faith, were suspected of colluding with ISIS to identify women to be targeted. These barriers to return home, raised by their faith, had to be addressed in the project through work with local religious leaders who took a lead role in finding solutions to convince community members to respect and reintegrate the returning women sur-

---

[14] See https://www.unodc.org/pdf/criminal_justice/UN_Rules_for_the_Treatment_of_Women_Prisoners_and_non-custodial_Measures_for_Women_Offenders_Bangkok_Rules.pdf

[15] See https://www.ohchr.org/en/statements/2022/11/international-day-women-human-rights-defenders-statement-united-nations-high

vivors. Despite this, many women choose to remain in "safe" camps to hide their "shame" (Kizilhan, Steger, et al., 2020), and suffer from extreme psychological trauma.

In response to this, the international team working on this project, headed by Professor Kizilhan, organized a rapid extraction project. This project brought female Yazidi survivors of ISIS abduction and abuse to Germany and into a support program. This was provided in a safe country with rapid and unbureaucratic support of the German government, in addition to capacity building and local projects in their home country (Beckmann et al., 2022; Kizilhan & Wenzel, 2020). This example highlights the need for unorthodox, rapid interventions that may be necessary in certain situations. Relocation, despite its controversy, is sometimes the best solution in a crisis, to provide immediate security and aid in the recovery of victims of extreme trauma. Changing perceptions and cultural models can be a slow process within origin countries with gender-biased environments.

The impact of mass violence as a challenge to public healthcare systems

The impact of war and mass violence affects individuals, groups, societies, and health systems as a whole. Therefore, this must be approached as a multilevel challenge when developing projects in war areas, such as northern Iraq.

As we will demonstrate through the description of the pilot project, interventions must be interdisciplinary and multi-level in nature. These interventions should utilize sustainable strategies that are likely to be continued by local stakeholders and teams, especially after international support fades out and shifts to address other emerging crisis areas.

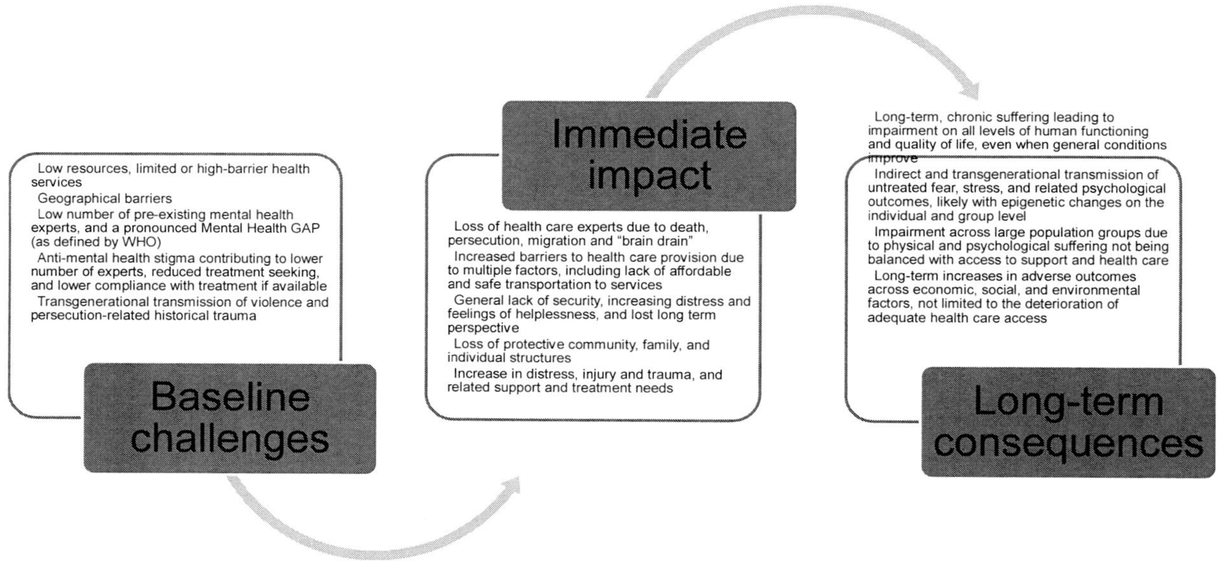

Fig. 1-2 Impact of historical and cultural mass violence on public health care systems and mental health[16]

[16] Reproduced with permission by the authors, from: Oxford Handbook on Violence, Oxford University Press 2024 (in print)

At baseline, before the beginning of atrocities imposed by war and conflict, healthcare systems already face considerable challenges, including low resources, a limited number of trained mental health professionals, geographic and economic barriers to treatment, and unequal access to services for different groups. Stigma against mental health as a health topic, and also against mental health patients and mental health care experts, is also an issue.

From the outset, the limited number of available local healthcare experts in countries like Iraq may have been killed, imprisoned, or forced to flee the country to safer regions, contributing to a "brain drain" of professionals. Only a small number of healthcare professionals may be able to hold out. In addition, it can become more difficult and more dangerous for people to travel to the few service providers left, who may also be overwhelmed and understaffed, as acts of mass violence lead to suffering and distress, especially, but not only, in those already vulnerable and underserved. This can be further aggravated by the interruption or loss of protective factors such as family and community networks. International support efforts may face the same problems and are often neither culture-sensitive nor well-planned and sustainable.

The long-term consequences can be severe, with chronic suffering, increased vulnerability, and potential transgenerational transmission of suffering in large parts of the population (Kizilhan et al., 2023; Kizilhan et al., 2021). Healthcare services can be overwhelmed and not sufficiently staffed by competent experts, while alternative support structures will be slow in rebuilding. The "brain drain" of experts will be difficult to improve. Loss of experts in these settings might be worsened by lack of access to advanced learning and interrupted professional development due to bureaucracy.

As trauma treatment models are often the primary focus in post-conflict regions, we want to provide a short overview of psychological trauma models, treatment options, and support systems, and their fast development over the last decades. Before delving into this, we want to remind the reader not to lose track of the previously described multilevel impact of war and violence. This includes the well-documented WHO mental health (treatment) GAP ("Mental health: WHO minds the GAP," 2010), which remains a significant factor to consider in planning projects in war-torn areas.

History of trauma concepts

Understanding and diagnosing survivors who have been directly or indirectly affected by the previously described forms of violence and human rights violations, or researching the mental health impact of these extreme life events, is more challenging than it might appear at first glance. The diagnostic concept of post-traumatic stress disorder (PTSD) has been recently firmly established through a long and complex process, which we will summarize in this chapter. The development of PTSD as a diagnosis is significant not only in medicine but also for public understanding and most legal systems. However, it is important to approach this development with care, without underestimating the importance of this medical diagnosis.

There are two key issues we want to raise to keep in mind when researching or planning services for survivors of extreme violence. First, PTSD should not receive attention as the only psychological consequence of stress or violence (Penk & Robinowitz, 1989). Second, recent research has on the other hand demonstrated that the basic neuropsychological mechanisms of PTSD are ingrained in the human biological system, probably as a result of evolutionary adaptation to dangerous environments (Baldwin, 2013). In principle, it can therefore be seen as a normal reaction to extreme forms of stress, that is common across all humans and cultures. However, it is important to remember that culture significantly influences how symptoms are shaped and perceived within specific cultural environments. To gain a better understanding of this, we must look back at the history of how PTSD and reactions to extremely distressing life events have been understood in the broadest sense.

Posttraumatic stress in civilian populations

Historically, it was not clearly understood that extreme life events could have specific long-term psychological consequences, even in people without pre-existing vulnerabilities. Most historical accounts trace the beginning of the modern concept of posttraumatic stress to the first railway accidents around 1830. The symptoms were also described as "railway spine", a term proposed by the UK surgeon Erich Erichsen in 1866, who suggested that symptoms were caused by "concussion of the spine followed by molecular changes" (Harrington, 1996). While descriptions of symptoms in victims of these first railway accidents include what we might now recognize as symptoms of PTSD, many victims also suffered from symptoms we would today rather classify as somatoform or conversion symptoms. These are symptoms that cannot be completely explained by medically accepted physical mechanisms or by imaging technology. At the time, some authors, as shown by Fischer-Homberg (1970), suspected that victims' claims were motivated by potential financial compensation from railway companies. As a result, illness claims were often discredited or said to be based on fictitious symptoms. This tendency to dismiss victim's psychological suffering as exaggerations has a long history and, in our experience, persists even today (Barrash et al., 2007; Gold, 1998).

At the turn of the 20th century, leading innovators in psychology and psychiatry, notably Sigmund Freud, held ambivalent views about symptoms in their patients. Initially, they attributed symptoms to trauma caused by sexual abuse (Summit, 1989). This concept was later explored by Sandor Ferenczi (Gutierrez-Pelaez & Herrera-Pardo, 2017). Today, these symptoms are likely understood as conversion symptoms, that can respond positively to psychological treatments. However, if we follow the historical development, it is clear that the observation of a link between sexual trauma and later symptoms was not sufficiently pursued or widely accepted in the early days, both within the medical field and the general public, especially in sexual abuse victims (Summit, 1989).

The difficulty of demonstrating the well-established physical and neuropsychological aspects of PTSD in individual victims outside of research settings might contribute to challenges in legal contexts. This includes the brain systems involved in fear and memory, such as the amygdala and hippocampus (Woodward et al., 2006), and even potential anatomical changes in the hippocampus observed in long-term sufferers (Tischler et al., 2006). Challenges arise because demonstrating these aspects can be difficult outside specialized research environments. For example, such limitations can pose difficulties when a PTSD diagnosis has legal implications, such as in asylum cases or the prosecution of perpetrators. Determining appropriate redress and compensation for victims can also be challenging in these situations. Despite these challenges, current scientific knowledge allows us to conclude that post-traumatic stress and trauma spectrum disorders are established medical disorders also in civilians. This remains true even when considering the influence of cultural factors and other variables on how individuals and groups present their suffering.

Returning back to medical history, following the 1830 railway accidents, the next major historical event to highlight the psychological effects of extreme violence on civilians was the establishment of concentration camps by the Nazi regime as part of the Holocaust genocide. This period led to the rediscovery of the idea that extreme life events can cause severe long-term psychological suffering, even in those without any prior vulnerability. The reemergence of this discussion was significant for several reasons. It helped to inform the development of treatment approaches, improve understanding of the long-term consequences of violence, and helped to combat the stigma sometimes attached to survivors. This stigma can hinder their recovery and restoration of dignity.

As aptly expressed by Leo Eitinger, a pioneer in the so-called concentration camp survivor syndrome (CCSS), the impact of trauma can be profound and, if severe enough, intervene with recovery or any "posttraumatic growth". Eitinger said, "If you go with a bicycle through a meadow, a few leaves of grass will be broken and the others might recover but if you go with a bulldozer through the same meadow, all leaves of grass will be broken no matter how resilient"[17]. This critical remark, reflecting the discussion at that time, also introduces another important aspect which is discussed later in this chapter: post-traumatic growth (Peterson et al., 2008; Shakespeare-Finch & Enders, 2008). Post-traumatic growth, an indicator of positive coping following trauma, is often impossible after severe traumatic events due to the severity of trauma and adverse later environments.

During this period in medical history, the description and gradual acceptance of the existence of a CCSS was a major step forward (Niederland, 1981). This syndrome was recognized as a distinct condition, independent of factors like financial compensation claims, and categorized as a general medical condition for treatment and compensation purposes. It represented a significant shift from models like Rieger's earlier concept of "compensation neurosis" (Hausotter, 1996), which implied malingering.

This survivor syndrome was later included in the International Classification of Diseases 10th Edition (ICD-10) under the label F62.0 (Enduring personality change after catastrophic experience). However, this diagnosis was not adopted by the US American Diagnostic and Statistical Manual of Mental Disorders (DSM). It was ultimately removed from the new ICD-11, likely due to a lack of diagnostic instruments and research focused on this specific diagnosis. It should not be confused with a personality "disorder", as the personality changes associated with CCSS develop as a direct result of the impact of extreme trauma, after an individual's personality development has already reached a certain stage. From the outset, the range of symptoms and underlying psychological or biological mechanisms have been the focus of research and discussion. Even some of the first authors describing symptoms of the concentration camp survivors attributed symptoms to physical factors like malnutrition or brain injury.

---

[17] Leo Eitinger, personal communication

However, experienced authors like Leo Eitinger emphasized a different perspective (Eitinger, 1961, 1962), pioneering the understanding of symptoms as natural or normal reactions to an extreme, abnormal event.

This complex history highlights the need for an open mind regarding the symptoms observed in survivors of extreme violence, war, and torture. While it is generally accepted that psychological stress is the main factor in trauma-related illness and might require special diagnostic and treatment considerations, blunt brain injury should also be seen as a common problem in violence, including war-related events. Post-concussional syndrome might be overlooked or neglected in at least some survivors due to a one-sided, singular focus on PTSD, especially as symptoms such as concentration difficulties partly overlap or might interact with PTSD symptoms (Shandera-Ochsner et al., 2013; Tanev et al., 2014; Wisco et al., 2014; Yeh et al., 2014).

Ettinger attributed the delay in reporting comprehensive data after World War II (WWII) to the different issues preoccupying researchers directly after the war. Another reason for the delay might be the lack of international standardization and agreement on definitions, concepts, and criteria in a time of "national" schools of psychiatry. Further, research on soldiers and civilians diverged, prompting some researchers to explore the concept of "war sailor syndrome," given war sailors were civilians thrust into a military war environment and faced challenges in gaining recognition and compensation (Sorensen et al., 1983).

Further categories like "Acute stress reaction" (also explored as a reaction in helpers (Soldatos et al., 2006)) and "Adjustment disorders" have been included in diagnostic classifications and manuals (Casey, 2014), but with less clear conceptual models and criteria. It is not clear whether they will be included as illnesses or medical disorders in future revisions of these classifications and manuals. Acute stress (disorder) might be relevant as it might predict the later development of PTSD, especially if dissociative symptoms that might inhibit coping are present (Brewin et al., 1999).

Posttraumatic stress in non-civilian populations

Historically, traumatic stress has received special consideration in the context of war, with war-related trauma in soldiers being a well-documented issue. This remains an important concern in war zones today. Early concepts of war-related trauma in soldiers included the "soldier's heart" (Engel, 2004; Jones, 2006; Troiani, 2012), which was documented after the US Civil War and in other conflicts. However, several important caveats exist. Authors like Derek Summerfield already have from early on drawn attention to the fact that PTSD symptoms must be considered within the context of culture. PTSD symptoms might not always be the most relevant problem for victims in a specific culture (Summerfield, 1991, 1998), and ICD and DSM PTSD categories might be seen as "Western cultural constructs" (Summerfield, 2002), despite the earlier mentioned universal biological mechanisms. Moreover, certain "subcultures" which are specific to a group, military unit, or country might also influence the development of symptoms, coping strategies, and the services that are offered. Further, special confounding problems like the already mentioned blunt brain injuries resulting from exposure to blasts (Colamaria et al., 2022; Rosenfeld & Ford, 2010) should also be considered in diagnostical and treatment considerations. They are not only a threat to soldiers but may also affect civilians and children in terrorist attacks (Singh et al., 2014) involving the prohibited use of cluster bombs and other wide-impact materials in war areas (Fares et al., 2014).

When again examining the historical developments in medicine and psychology, particularly regarding the long term impact of war, we see that World War I (WW) had a profound effect. Many soldiers who survived the extreme horrors of trench warfare were often unprepared young persons, confronted with technologically advanced weaponry and unprecedented warfare situations. The medical literature of the time documented the new category of "Kriegszitterer" (Peckl, 2007) (best translated as "persons with war-related trembling disorder"). This term, along with "shell-shock" (Crocq & Crocq, 2000; Dayan & Olliac, 2010; Shively & Perl, 2012), was well-known to military psychiatrists and the public, due to extensive documentation in visual materials from that era. Depending on the belief system of the treating doctor, this condition was seen as either an illness out of the control of the patient, and as a reason for concern, support, respect, and treatment, or as a sign of weakness, or even as an attempt to escape the war as a defector. Treatment efforts at that time consequently ranged from support and protection to rather violent forms of treatment, such as electroshock "treatment" or even execution as a defector.

The existence of an accepted medical category later provided protection against discrimination within medical systems that were likely strongly influenced by racist concepts at the time, and promoted by figures of the medical establishment who continued to adhere to fascist ideologies supporting stigmatizing interpretations even after the war (Ernst, 1996, 1997), without consequences. The efforts of these medical personalities to discredit survivors, and dismiss the psychological impacts of extreme violence and human rights violations as mere inventions of survivors or biased medical experts, were partially successful. This was seen in the case of the resistance against the aforementioned "survivor syndrome", which created additional suffering in the victims and has been observed firsthand in our practice with survivors.

It may be a consequence of these historical barriers that it took a considerable amount of time until the direct connection between extreme life events, distress, and long-term psychological suffering was firmly established in medical systems. A first category, termed "gross stress reaction", which was observed in survivors of the Korean war (Shin & Yim, 2023) had been proposed in the US DSM (Diagnostical and Statistical Manual) in version I, but was consequently abandoned. This was followed by a complex history of changes in the diagnostic criteria, reflecting a growing body of research on the "new" disorder, up to the US DSM III revision around 1980 (Kim, 2012; Wilson, 1994). Several authors have explored the development and implementation of the concept of PTSD as the first clear stress, or trauma-related, serious medical condition (Kim, 2012; Wilson, 1994). They have drawn attention to the suffering of Vietnam War veterans who, with the help of a supporting group of medical doctors and survivor organizations, ensured the inclusion of the concept in the standard manual (see Shay, 1994 for a detailed description).

Child soldiers

At this point, we wish to address the complexities experienced by child soldiers. They are a special group of survivors that are frequently neglected, but are of great relevance in countries like also Iraq. Gary Humpreys, an expert in this area, reports that while "a United Nations treaty prohibiting the use of children in hostilities has been ratified by 126 countries…(but) at least 250 000 child soldiers are currently involved in armed conflicts worldwide" (Humphreys, 2009). The United Nations Children's Fund (UNICEF) and its partners are active in helping children in returning to a normal life. Psychological trauma is common in these children, who are frequently victims of abduction, indoctrination, and torture before becoming soldiers, and then often perpetrators of atrocities (Somasundaram, 2002). In a study of Yazidi children who had been abducted and used as child soldiers in Iraq, Kizilhan and Noll-Hussong (2018) reported that the children showed significantly higher prevalence of PTSD (48.3%), depressive disorders (45.6%), anxiety disorders (45.8%) and somatic disturbances (50.6%), compared to boys who had not been child soldiers in a control group. The authors also reported that "developmentally crucial self-esteem was significantly reduced in former child soldiers" (Kizilhan & Noll-Hussong, 2018). Research has even examined the fate of child soldiers in industrialized countries, like Germany. For example, studies of German WWII veteran children showed lower rates of PTSD as compared to the children from the Iraq sample, probably reflecting the better post-war conditions in Germany or different methodology (Kuwert, Knaevelsrud, et al., 2008; Kuwert, Spitzer, et al., 2008). Most recently, we observed the use of child soldiers in Uganda, where they were abducted, brainwashed, and tortured by Josef Konys LRA terrorist group (Amone-P'Olak et al., 2014; Klasen et al., 2015; Vindevogel et al., 2013).

The rehabilitation needs of child soldiers are complex and might require culturally-sensitive approaches in the communities where the children are located after the conflict (Betancourt, 2008, 2010; Betancourt et al., 2013; Betancourt et al., 2008), and where they often struggle with stigma (Betancourt et al., 2010) and confused identities. The reactions of their original communities upon their return differ widely. Some children will experience stigma-based isolation, while others will experience a slow acceptance and vigorous efforts to reintegrate them as valuable parts of the community, without punishing them for possible atrocities they might have committed as soldiers against civilians of the same or other communities.

Rehabilitation projects face many challenges, as observed for example by Betancourt et al. (2008) in Sierra Leone. A recent publication by Klasen et al. (2010) reported high rates of resilience in some groups of child soldiers, stating that "27.6% (of a group of former child soldiers) showed posttraumatic resilience as indicated by the absence of posttraumatic stress disorder, depression, and clinically significant behavioral and emotional problems" (Klasen, Oettingen, Daniels, & Adam, 2010; Klasen, Oettingen, Daniels, Post, et al., 2010). The authors also drew attention to the need for further research to better understand and conceptualize developmental trauma disorder after experiences of severe trauma in childhood, which interrupts normal development. Transitional justice might be necessary in some post-conflict settings to facilitate reintegration.

Posttraumatic growth and resilience

Posttraumatic growth and the development of resilience, as noted by Agaibi and Wilson (2005), are not commonly expected if a traumatic event is severe enough, as noted before. However, since the first pioneer publications by Werner (2012) on war children, numerous studies have explored, if and how individuals exposed to difficult life experiences cope. Both posttraumatic growth and resilience can be seen as helpful variations of "good" coping strategies that can be supported by MHPSS, specific interventions, or by "Positive Psychotherapy", the latter having been applied in Iraq (Kizilhan & Wenzel, 2020). They are important as counter-strategies to a one-sided focus on illness and suffering, and are part of the related concept of "salutogenesis", which has been promoted for example by Antonovsky (see Antonovsky, 2022). Resilience, the capacity to recover after difficult events, might have genetic (Sarapas et al., 2011) and early imprinting factors, but can also be learned and promoted, which is an important lesson for war areas, if you want to promote posttraumatic growth. Resilience can describe coping in different situations, ranging from individual or communal challenges, to health crises and environmental, social, and historical changes. Resilience is also the focus of several recent EU projects[18].

Recent research has begun to identify neurobiological aspects of resilience, besides genetic factors. For example, links between Interferon Gamma and Interleukin factors have been shown in Vietnam war veterans (Bruenig et al., 2018) and on the role of Oxytocin (Sippel et al., 2017), underlining the importance of physical factors in the better understanding of resilience. Other authors have underlined the importance of (perceived) social support (Panagioti et al., 2014). However, it might be too early to propose an integrated model that explains how psychological coping and neurobiological changes contribute to positive outcomes in difficult situations. Resilience and posttraumatic growth may be stronger indicators to use in research on interventions for trauma spectrum disorders, and might predict better long-term outcomes, than measures which only demonstrate a reduction in trauma symptoms. New models, such as the use of online tools to build resilience[19], may also be used in war areas and areas with a challenging infrastructure. These tools were also used in the pilot project in Iraq (Wagner et al., 2012).

PTSD as it is presently defined in the WHO's ICD-11 handbook

Below, we cite the full text for the ICD-11 definition of PTSD[20] due to the importance of the concept. Given the rapid development of medical concepts and knowledge, it is important to use diagnostic criteria with care in clinical practice. We believe the ICD-11 description is better structured and more adequate in reflecting research and clinical observations than the US–DSM model, which is popular in most international research projects.

---

[18] See the authors project at http://www.resilience-project.eu/
[19] See again http://www.resilience-project.eu/
[20] https://icd.who.int/en

ICD definitions are part of a more comprehensive health assessment of not only mental but also physical illness, and are supported by the World Health Organization (WHO) as a global standard. The WHO has also developed an "International Classification of Functioning, Disability and Health" (ICF) to describe the impact of symptoms in a public health-oriented model, which has been tested in refugee groups (Jorgensen et al., 2010). The ICF could be used together with diagnostical models.

"Code: 6B40 Posttraumatic stress disorder

Description

Post-traumatic stress disorder (PTSD) may develop following exposure to an extremely threatening or horrific event or series of events. It is characterized by all of the following: 1) re-experiencing the traumatic event or events in the present in the form of vivid intrusive memories, flashbacks, or nightmares. Re-experiencing may occur via one or multiple sensory modalities and is typically accompanied by strong or overwhelming emotions, particularly fear or horror, and strong physical sensations; 2) avoidance of thoughts and memories of the event or events, or avoidance of activities, situations, or people reminiscent of the event(s); and 3) persistent perceptions of heightened current threat, for example as indicated by hypervigilance or an enhanced startle reaction to stimuli such as unexpected noises. The symptoms persist for at least several weeks and cause significant impairment in personal, family, social, educational, occupational or other important areas of functioning.

Inclusions: Traumatic neurosis
Exclusions: Acute stress reaction (QE84), Complex post traumatic stress disorder(6B41)

Matching Terms *PTSD* - [post traumatic stress disorder]

Diagnostic Requirements

Essential (Required) Features:

- Exposure to an event or situation (either short- or long-lasting) of an extremely threatening or horrific nature. Such events include, but are not limited to, directly experiencing natural or human-made disasters, combat, serious accidents, torture, sexual violence, terrorism, assault or acute life-threatening illness (e.g., a heart attack);

witnessing the threatened or actual injury or death of others in a sudden, unexpected, or violent manner; and learning about the sudden, unexpected or violent death of a loved one.

- Following the traumatic event or situation, the development of a characteristic syndrome lasting for at least several weeks, consisting of all three core elements:
- Re-experiencing the traumatic event in the present, in which the event(s) is not just remembered but is experienced as occurring again in the here and now. This typically occurs in the form of vivid intrusive memories or images; flashbacks, which can vary from mild (there is a transient sense of the event occurring again in the present) to severe (there is a complete loss of awareness of present surroundings), or repetitive dreams or nightmares that are thematically related to the traumatic event(s). Re-experiencing is typically accompanied by strong or overwhelming emotions, such as fear or horror, and strong physical sensations. Re-experiencing in the present can also involve feelings of being overwhelmed or immersed in the same intense emotions that were experienced during the traumatic event, without a prominent cognitive aspect, and may occur in response to reminders of the event. Reflecting on or ruminating about the event(s) and remembering the feelings that one experienced at that time are not sufficient to meet the re-experiencing requirement.
- Deliberate avoidance of reminders likely to produce re-experiencing of the traumatic event(s). This may take the form either of active internal avoidance of thoughts and memories related to the event(s), or external avoidance of people, conversations, activities, or situations reminiscent of the event(s). In extreme cases the person may change their environment (e.g., move to a different city or change jobs) to avoid reminders.
- Persistent perceptions of heightened current threat, for example as indicated by hypervigilance or an enhanced startle reaction to stimuli such as unexpected noises. Hypervigilant persons constantly guard themselves against danger and feel themselves or others close to them to be under immediate threat either in specific situations or more generally. They may adopt new behaviours designed to ensure safety (e.g., not sitting with ones' back to the door, repeated checking in vehicles' rear-view mirrors).
- The disturbance results in significant impairment in personal, family, social, educational, occupational or other important areas of functioning. If functioning is maintained, it is only through significant additional effort.

Additional Clinical Features:

- Common symptomatic presentations of Post-Traumatic Stress Disorder may also include general dysphoria, dissociative symptoms, somatic complaints, suicidal ideation and behaviour, social withdrawal, excessive alcohol or drug use to avoid re-experiencing or manage emotional reactions, anxiety symptoms including panic, and obsessions or compulsions in response to memories or reminders of the trauma.
- The emotional experience of individuals with Post-Traumatic Stress Disorder commonly includes anger, shame, sadness, humiliation, or guilt, including survivor guilt.

Boundary with Normality (Threshold):

- A history of exposure to an event or situation of an extremely threatening or horrific nature does not in itself indicate the presence of Post-Traumatic Stress Disorder. Many people experience such stressors without developing a disorder. Rather, the presentation must meet all diagnostic requirements for the disorder.

Course Features:

- Onset of Post-Traumatic Stress Disorder can occur at any time during the life span following exposure to a traumatic event.
- Onset of Post-Traumatic Stress Disorder symptoms typically occurs within three months following exposure to a traumatic event. However, delays in the expression of Post-Traumatic Stress Disorder symptomology can occur even years after exposure to a traumatic event.
- The symptoms and course of Post-Traumatic Stress Disorder can vary significantly over time and individuals. Recurrence of symptoms may occur after to exposure to reminders of the traumatic event or as a result of experiencing additional life stressors or traumatic events. Some individuals diagnosed with Post-Traumatic Stress Disorder can experience persistent symptoms for months or years without reprieve.
- Nearly one half of individuals diagnosed with Post-Traumatic Stress Disorder will experience complete recovery of symptoms within 3 months of onset.

Developmental Presentations:

- Post-Traumatic Stress Disorder can occur at all ages, but responses to a traumatic event—that is, the core elements of the characteristic syndrome—manifest differently depending on age and developmental stage.
- Emerging cognitive capacities and limited verbal abilities for self-report in young children (e.g., less than 6 years of age) makes it more difficult to assess for the presence of re-experiencing, active avoidance of internal states, and perceptions of heightened current threat. Assessments of symptoms should not be based exclusively on child-reported internal symptoms but include caregiver reports of observable behavioural symptoms emerging after traumatic experiences.
- In younger children, evidence of the core symptoms supporting a diagnosis of Post-Traumatic Stress Disorder often manifests behaviourally, such as in trauma-specific reenactments that may occur during repetitive play or in drawings, frightening dreams without clear content or night terrors, or uncharacteristic impulsivity. However, children may not necessarily appear distressed when talking about or playing out their traumatic recollections, despite substantial impact on psychosocial functioning and development. Other manifestations of Post-Traumatic Stress Disorder in pre-school children may be less trauma-specific and include both inhibited and disinhibited behaviours. For example, hypervigilance may manifest as increased frequency and intensity of temper tantrums, separation anxiety, regression in skills (e.g., verbal skills, toileting), exaggerated age-associated fears, or excessive crying. External avoidance or expressions of recollection of traumatic experiences may be evidenced by a new onset of acting out, protective or rescue strategies, limited exploration or reluctance to engage in new activities, and excessive reassurance seeking from a trusted caregiver.
- Limited capacity to reflect on and report internal states may also be characteristic of some school-age children and adolescents. Furthermore, children and adolescents may be more reluctant than adults to report their reactions to traumatic events. In such cases, greater reliance on changes in behaviour such as increased trauma-specific reenactments or overt avoidance may be necessary.
- Children or adolescents may deny feelings of distress or horror associated with re-experiencing but rather report no affect or other

types of strong or overwhelming emotions as a part of re-experiencing, including those that are non-distressing.

- In adolescence, reluctance to pursue developmental opportunities (e.g., to gain autonomy from caregivers) may be a sign of psychosocial impairment. Self-injurious or risky behaviours (e.g., substance use or unprotected sex) occur at elevated rates among adolescents and adults with Post-Traumatic Stress Disorder.
- Assessment can be complicated in children and adolescents when loss of a parent or caregiver is associated with a traumatic event or an intervention. For example, a chronically abused child who is removed from the home may place greater emphasis on the loss of a primary caregiver than on aspects of the experience that might objectively be considered more threatening or horrific.
- Among older adults with Post-Traumatic Stress Disorder, symptom severity may decline over the life course, especially re-experiencing. However, avoidance of situations, people, activities, or conversations about the event(s) as well as hypervigilance typically persist. Older persons may dismiss their symptoms as a normal part of life, which may be related to shame and fear of stigma.

Culture-Related Features:

- The salience of particular Post-Traumatic Stress Disorder symptoms may vary across cultures. For example, in some groups anger may be the most prominent symptom related to traumatic exposure, and the most culturally appropriate way of expressing distress. In other cultural contexts, nightmares may have elaborated cultural significance that increases their importance in assessing for the characteristic symptoms of Post-Traumatic Stress Disorder.
- Symptoms central to Post-Traumatic Stress Disorder in some cultures may not be included in descriptions of the disorder and may therefore be missed by clinicians unfamiliar with those cultural expressions. For example, somatic symptoms such as headaches (often with visual aura), dizziness, bodily heat, shortness of breath, gastrointestinal distress, trembling, and orthostatic hypotension may be prominent.
- Cultural variation may affect Post-Traumatic Stress Disorder onset and the meaning of traumatic stressors. For example, some cultural groups attribute greater risk of Post-Traumatic Stress Disorder to traumatic events affecting family members than the person him/herself; other societies may find it particularly traumatic to ob-

serve the desecration or destruction of religious symbols or to be denied the ability to perform funeral rites for deceased relatives.
- Certain trauma-related symptoms may be associated with intense fear in particular cultural contexts, due to their connection with specific catastrophic cognitions, and may precipitate panic attacks in the context of Post-Traumatic Stress Disorder. These catastrophic interpretations may impact the trajectory of the disorder and be associated with greater severity, chronicity or poorer response to treatment. For example, some Latin American patients may consider trauma-related trembling to be the precursor of a lifelong condition of severe *nervios* (nerves) and some Cambodians may interpret palpitations as signs of a 'weak heart.'
- Some Post-Traumatic Stress Disorder symptoms may not be viewed as pathological in some cultural groups. For example, intrusive thoughts may be considered normal rather than a symptom indicating illness. It is important to evaluate the presence of all required diagnostic elements including functional impairment rather than treating any one symptom as pathognomonic.

Sex- and/or Gender-Related Features:

- Post-Traumatic Stress Disorder is more common among females.
- Females diagnosed with Post-Traumatic Stress Disorder are more likely to experience a longer duration of impairment and higher levels of negative emotionality and somatic symptoms as a part of their clinical presentation.

Boundaries with Other Disorders and Conditions (Differential Diagnosis):

- *Boundary with Complex Post-Traumatic Stress Disorder:* Whereas the diagnostic requirements for Complex Post-Traumatic Stress Disorder include all Essential Features of Post-Traumatic Stress Disorder, the diagnosis of Complex Post-Traumatic Stress Disorder also requires the additional Essential Features of severe problems in affect regulation, persistent negative beliefs about oneself, and persistent difficulties in sustaining relationships.
- *Boundary with Prolonged Grief Disorder:* Similar to Post-Traumatic Stress Disorder, Prolonged Grief Disorder may occur in individuals who experience bereavement as a result of the death of a loved one occurring in traumatic circumstances. In Post-Traumatic Stress Disorder, where the individual re-experiences the event or situation associated with the death, in Prolonged Grief

Disorder the person may be preoccupied with memories of the circumstances surrounding the death but, unlike in Post-Traumatic Stress Disorder, does not re-experience them as occurring again in the here and now.

- *Boundary with Adjustment Disorder:* In Adjustment Disorder, the stressor can be of any severity or any type, and is not necessarily of an extremely threatening or horrific nature. A response to a less serious event or situation that otherwise meets the symptom requirements for Post-Traumatic Stress Disorder but that is beyond the duration appropriate for Acute Stress Reaction should be diagnosed as Adjustment Disorder. Moreover, many people who experience an extremely threatening or horrific event develop symptoms that do not meet the full diagnostic requirements for Post-Traumatic Stress Disorder; these reactions are generally better diagnosed as Adjustment Disorder.
- *Boundary with Acute Stress Reaction:* Normal acute reactions to traumatic events can include all the symptoms of Post-Traumatic Stress Disorder including re-experiencing, but these begin to subside fairly quickly (e.g., within 1 week after the event terminates or removal from the threatening situation, or 1 month in the case of ongoing stressors). If clinical intervention is warranted in these situations, a diagnosis of Acute Stress Reaction from the chapter on 'Factors Influencing Health Status or Contact with Health Services' (i.e., a non-disorder category) is generally most appropriate.
- *Boundary with Schizophrenia or Other Primary Psychotic Disorders:* Some individuals with Post-Traumatic Stress Disorder re-experience traumatic events in the form of severe flashbacks that may have a hallucinatory quality or are hypervigilant to threat to the extent that they may appear to be paranoid. Auditory pseudo-hallucinations, recognized as being the person's own thoughts and of internal origin, can occur in Post-Traumatic Stress Disorder. Such symptoms should not be considered evidence of a psychotic disorder.
- *Boundary with Depressive Episode:* In a Depressive Episode, intrusive memories are not experienced as occurring again in the present, but as belonging to the past, and they are often accompanied by rumination. However, Depressive Episodes commonly co-occur with Post-Traumatic Stress Disorder, and an additional Mood Disorder diagnosis should be assigned if warranted.
- *Boundary with Panic Disorder:* In Post-Traumatic Stress Disorder, panic attacks can be triggered by reminders of the traumatic event(s) or in the context of re-experiencing. Panic attacks that oc-

cur entirely in these contexts do not warrant an additional, separate diagnosis of Panic Disorder. Instead, the 'with panic attacks' specifier (MB23.H) may be applied. However, if unexpected panic attacks (i.e., those that come on 'out of the blue') are also present and the other diagnostic requirements are met, an additional diagnosis of Panic Disorder is appropriate.

- Boundary with Specific Phobia: In some cases, a situational or conditioned Specific Phobia can arise after exposure to a traumatic event (e.g., being attacked by a dog). Specific Phobia can generally be differentiated from Post-Traumatic Stress Disorder by the absence of re-experiencing of the event in the present. Although phobic responses may include powerful memories of the event, in response to which the individual experiences anxiety, the memories are experienced as belonging to the past.
- *Boundary with Dissociative Disorders:* Following an experience of a traumatic event(s), a variety of dissociative symptoms can occur, including somatic symptoms, memory disturbances, flashbacks or other trance-like states, alterations in identity and sense of agency, and experiences of depersonalization, especially during the episodes of re-experiencing. If the dissociative symptoms are confined to episodes of re-experiencing in an individual with Post-Traumatic Stress Disorder or Complex Post-Traumatic Stress Disorder, an additional diagnosis of a Dissociative Disorder should not be assigned. If significant dissociative symptoms are present outside of episodes of re-experiencing and the full diagnostic requirements are met, an additional Dissociative Disorder diagnosis may be assigned.
- *Boundary with other mental disorders:* It is common for other mental disorders other than or in addition to Post-Traumatic Stress Disorder to develop in the aftermath of an event or situation (either short- or long-lasting) of an extremely threatening or horrific nature. Thus, a history of exposure to a potentially traumatic event does not in itself indicate the presence of Post-Traumatic Stress Disorder. Depressive Disorders, Anxiety or Fear-Related Disorders, Disorders Due to Substance Use, and Dissociative Disorders can all occur in the aftermath of potentially traumatic experiences, often in the absence of Post-Traumatic Stress Disorder.“ (Note: end of quote)

The definition illustrates how complex the PTSD model has become. Qualitative research might be advisable when exploring PTSD symptoms in a new setting or culture, keeping up with changing definitions (Wenzel et al., 2015) and upcoming new research.

PTSD and culture

An important lesson from the arguments raised by Summerfield in the seventies, and by others in the following years, is the recognition that trauma-related symptoms are perceived and presented in different forms in different cultural contexts, following severe life events. In European "Western" cultures, this shift can be seen in the disappearance of conversion symptoms, which occurred as medical culture and society evolved earlier as a common problem after traumatic events and before recent diagnostical tools and models. These symptoms have been arguably replaced by the recognition of PTSD as both a medically and socially accepted issue. While these changes in Western cultures could be seen as a transcultural phenomenon, it also became clear that symptom profiles, interpretation, and focus on symptoms by individuals and society became an issue in the rapidly developing field of transcultural psychiatry (as promoted by Summerfield).

The next major paradigm shift regarding PTSD and culture was probably the increased inclusion of cultural factors in the US-dominated DSM, which was widely used in many countries (especially for research). This began with the somewhat tentative inclusion of specific "culture-bound syndromes" (Keshavan, 2014; Ventriglio et al., 2016), like "Latah". These inclusions might be seen as a lingering echo of quasi-colonialist fascination with rare and unusual phenomena in "primitive" cultures. Other researchers, such as Kleinman, developed models to include culture and culture-related aspects of illness and suffering in public health models (as discussed below, see also Borisova et al., 2017). Kizilhan, the leader of our Iraq project, has explored diverse aspects of culture, including the difference between psychotherapy in collectivistic, group-oriented societies and in individualistic societies (Kizilhan, 2014).

Kleinman, a pioneer in this field, in turn challenged concepts of what should be described as an "*illness*" or as a "*disease*". While the two terms are often used interchangeably, they are viewed quite differently through a cultural anthropology approach. Illness is defined as the "innately human experience of symptoms and suffering" (Hankoff, 1988).

This development was incorporated into the "cultural formulation outline" (Novins et al., 1997), and further refined in the DSM-5. Aggarwal (2023) proposed using an "intersubjective model of culture" through which patients and clinicians work collaboratively to navigate cultural similarities and differences. This highlights the shift in focus from the DSM-IV, to the most recent DSM-5 TR, which emphasizes global dynamic changes in cultures. This is particularly relevant in war areas. The "Cultural Formulation Interview" (CFI) is a freely available attachment to the

DSM-5, to help teach these concepts in the context of transcultural Psychiatry (Lam et al., 2023). However, more work is needed (Mezzich et al., 1999) as a short list of "official" DSM Cultural Concepts of Distress is not sufficient.

The "Criterium A" challenge and other challenges when assessing PTSD in research in war regions

The challenge of assessing PTSD in research in war regions is an ongoing controversy in the field. The DSM criteria includes a "Criterium A", which requires a triggering event for PTSD to be of significant severity (Fabra, 2003). This criterium was revised across multiple editions of the DSM, potentially with the aim of avoiding overdiagnosis of PTSD in research and clinical practice. However, research over the last few decades has demonstrated that a wide range of everyday life events, like a complicated birth experienced by a civilian (Anderson & McCarley, 2013; Yates et al., 2022), can trigger symptoms of PTSD. As previously described, this has been confirmed by the development of neurobiological and evolutionary models of the brain (Cantor, 2009), which describe PTSD as a fundamental process embedded in all brains, which evolved as a helpful mechanism for survival in subjectively dangerous situations. This information can also be important for educating PTSD patients, to address their insecurity and stigma, and to support them in the uptake of adequate treatment. It is further relevant for forensic assessments and can explain the high prevalence of PTSD symptoms linked to multiple traumatic events in war and post-conflict areas, as seen in Iraq. It is important to note that objective or retrospective assessments of the threat level should not be made by physicians alone. Rather, the patient's subjective level of perceived threat will determine their reactions, which is often neglected in the discussion. Events that create a high amount of shame (McCann et al., 2023), because of the fear of a "social" death, which might not objectively be followed by physical death, can also lead to PTSD and other reactive problems.

Most PTSD-focused questionnaires and diagnostic instruments avoid this problem by omitting any standardized measure of the events and the stress they have caused on a subjective level. This creates a problem in the literature on quantitative and epidemiological PTSD research. The Harvard Trauma Questionnaire (HTQ), which is popular in research, tries to address this problem by providing a special list of characteristics and potentially traumatic events which are relevant to the environment in which the research is taking place. This excellent questionnaire is continuously revised to list characteristics and events which fit other specific settings, such as the Hmong ethnic group and their war experiences. The questionnaire has also been recently upgraded to fit the experiences of refugee populations and to align with DSM-5 criteria (Berthold et al., 2019). From our perspective, most authors using this questionnaire do not conduct necessary preparatory research to identify events which could be experienced in new settings and cultures where they apply the questionnaire. They also rarely publish and validate their translations.

Structured instruments like the Clinician-Administered PTSD Scale for DSM-5 (CAPS-5) (Resick et al., 2023)[21] and The Structured Clinical Interview for DSM-5 (SCID)[22] interview schedules (Elhai et al., 2008; Zawadzki et al., 2015) include PTSD modules and might combine them with non-standardized modules for events. The increasing number of diagnostic instruments for PTSD further demonstrates the recent acceptance of PTSD as a diagnosis. Differences in diagnostic criteria between different DSM versions, APA DSM, and the WHOs ICD (Wenzel et al., 2015), as well as differences across cultures, still introduce challenges in getting reliable results.

Assessing PTSD is especially challenging in war and post-conflict areas, and in countries with diverse traditional cultures and low-income health systems. There are several reasons these challenges exist in this context:

1) In rapidly developing and emergency situations, selecting, acquiring, and adapting standard instruments as fast as is necessary can be difficult. Using a questionnaire might require permissions, access to the right language versions (if available), agreement on a specific scoring strategy (often there are several), and on getting funding for copyrighted commercialized instruments.

2) The cultural adaptation of an instrument may be difficult and should ideally be based on additional research which has evaluated cultural factors and appropriateness. In many situations, questionnaires with unclear validation status, or those which have just been adapted by the popular translation-retranslation method, have been used with large population samples. More recently, guidelines for a stricter procedure, which is less prone to errors during the translation-retranslation method, have been published and used (Larsson et al., 2007). Further, almost all commonly

[21] See https://www.ptsd.va.gov/professional/assessment/adult-int/caps.asp

[22] See https://www.appi.org/products/structured-clinical-interview-for-dsm-5-scid-

used instruments do not cover idioms of distress, which are culturally specific ways in which individuals express and communicate their psychological suffering and emotional problems. These are especially important in traditional societies with specific health belief models.

3) Questionnaires often only cover PTSD, or a limited range of possible disorders are considered. Published research demonstrates that in addition to PTSD, other reactive mental health problems, such as depression (Stompe et al., 2001; Wenzel et al., 2000), are also common and might need to be the more critical areas of focus.

4) The aforementioned criterion A problem is the last challenge we present and take up again. Events experienced in specific situations might differ, and there is a need for preparatory research to be conducted to identify and structure these events adequately. Language is important here; the word "torture," for example, can mean different things for non-legal professionals in different societies (Basoglu, 2009), independent from the UN definition. For example, in a survey we conducted after the war in Sarajevo, we discovered that exposure to propaganda that was maligning them was experienced as "torture" by many Bosnians.

Idioms of distress, health belief models, and cultural formulations

The wide range of cultures, each with their own illness behaviors, health belief models, and medical concepts, cannot be fully covered by a single handbook, even if we take it up again in this context. In transcultural interactions, it is crucial to have a deep understanding of each respective culture when planning and implementing support measures and psychotherapy (Beckmann et al., 2022; Kizilhan, 2014). This is especially important given the role these cultural factors play in the international application of the DSM-5 standard.

Forms of health belief models, describing what is believed about health, illness, and consequently treatment, in a culture or group, may be described as in Figure 1-3.

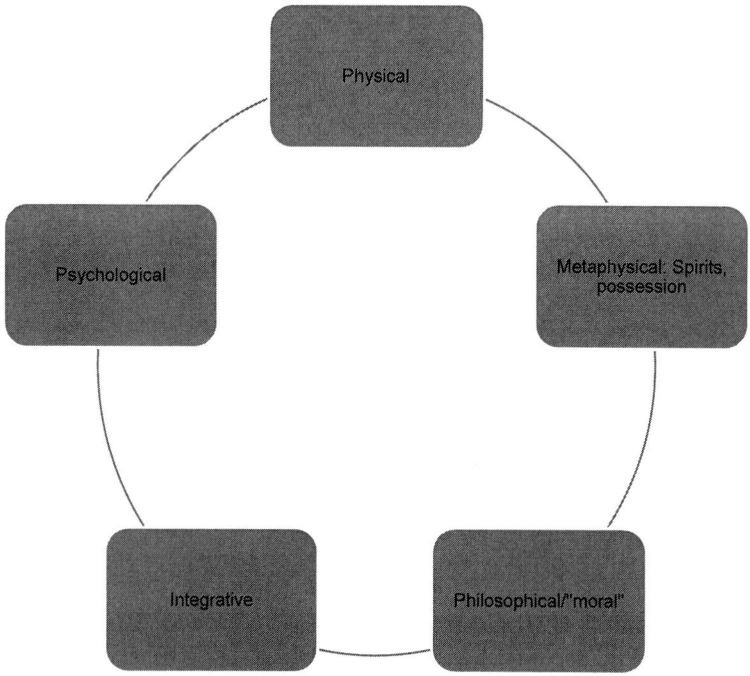

Fig. 1-3 Health belief models – a phenomenology

Some organizations aim to address this gap by creating detailed handbooks for understanding cultural formulations of distress in specific cultures. For instance, the UNHCR published an excellent handbook authored by Kirmayer and Hassan[23], which provides an overview of these issues for Syrian refugees. This handbook is available in both Arabic and Kurdish to reflect the different idioms of distress in both languages used in Syria.

Still, a lot of work is required in each different war and post-conflict zone, to identify and describe idioms of distress and cultural formulations that reflect the often highly diverse local cultures. This should not be forgotten in the use of questionnaires, even in emergency settings, as discussed separately in this chapter.

[23] Available from https://www.unhcr.org/media/culture-context-and-mental-health-and-psychosocial-wellbeing-syrians-review-mental-health-and

History of psychotherapy and approaches to treatment after extreme violence

Treatment models have in a similar way a longer history, as have concepts. They have been developed mostly by adapting existing evidence-based general treatment models, like Cognitive Behavior Therapy (CBT), to work in different cultures and for the needs of trauma victims. New techniques like Eye Movement Desensitization (EMDR) (Cukor et al., 2010; Raboni et al., 2006; Seidler & Wagner, 2006) or Narrative Exposure Therapy (NET) (Hensel-Dittmann et al., 2011) have also been added to the inventory of interventions available, and can also be used to supplement other treatment and support offers. Despite some controversy, the evidence base for these models is relatively firm, in contrast to the many, often experimental approaches, promoted in some war areas. For example, Hensel-Dittmann et al. (2011) for example compared 10 treatment sessions of NET with stress inoculation training (SIT) in a group of refugee war survivors in Germany. They found a significant decrease in PTSD symptoms (Hensel-Dittmann et al., 2011). It is open to debate whether these treatments can be used as "stand-alone" approaches or only within the framework of more established methods. Additionally, there is a question of whether health care professionals using these treatments should have a more comprehensive professional background, such as being trained psychotherapists or psychologists, as outlined in the curricula described later in this book. Further, when considering treatment outcomes, one may need to focus on a more complex range of indicators, such as quality of life and social and occupational functioning. There should be a long-term follow-up to evaluate if the results are stable over time, even under difficult circumstances.

In the use of psychopharmacological medications, it is important to give greater consideration to biological ethnic factors (Leung, 2023; Ruiz-White et al., 2023). These factors include not only cultural response patterns and stigma, but also differences in drug metabolism. Most pharmaceutical drugs are developed and primarily tested within a limited number of ethnic groups, in the US or Europe, which have diverse genetic, nutritional, and metabolic backgrounds (Ruiz-White et al., 2023).

Most advanced treatment models require the availability of a substantial number of highly trained and preferably local healthcare professionals. This issue is central in our pilot project presented in this book. The previously mentioned Cultural Formulation Interview (CFI) can be used to explore cultural aspects of mental health problems, prepare healthcare professionals for interactions with patients from other cultures (Skammeritz et al., 2020), and to modify treatment strategies. Trained experts are usually not available for larger displaced population groups, especially in developing countries, which requires long-term capacity building that considers all of the challenges we have outlined (Beckmann et al., 2022).

Mental health interventions in conflict and post-conflict environments

To address the outlined challenges and limitations, which are exacerbated by the impact of mass violence on various levels of health services, several strategies have been developed. These strategies offer necessary integrated and interdisciplinary approaches, which account for the specific challenges experienced prior to, during, or after mass violence. Community orientation has been, for example, pioneered by institutions like the Gaza Community Mental Health Project (Saymah et al., 2015).

The Mental Health and Psychosocial Services (MHPSS) model

Over the last few decades, leading international umbrella and UN organizations, including UNHCR, have developed and promoted the concept of Mental Health and Psychosocial Services (MHPSS), focusing mainly on low-resource, low barrier services that remain close to communities (see IASC Reference Group's (2010) book : "Mental Health and Psychosocial Support in Humanitarian Emergencies: What Should Humanitarian Health Actors Know?" and the Sphere Handbook's Standard on Mental Health (Sphere Project, 2018)[24]). MHPSS is discussed in more detail in it`s implementation in Iraq further down.

Other organizations, like the Dutch-based Transcultural Psychosocial Organization (TPO), have also pioneered similar concepts, likely with an even stronger focus on transcultural aspects of mental health. They have advocated for a special focus on the mental health impacts of violence and of displacement, considering these issues crucial within a comprehensive approach to culturally sensitive mental health in crisis and post-conflict settings[25].

---

[24] See https://spherestandards.org/wp-content/uploads/Sphere-Handbook-2018-EN.pdf

[25] https://www.healthnettpo.org/en/who-we-are

The MHPSS model, which is being increasingly endorsed by national governments (such as Germany[26]) and NGOs, typically promotes resilience-building, education, mutual and community support models, and stress-reduction strategies at various levels. It also takes into account factors like physical needs and safety, which can influence mental health, as seen in models such as the water, sanitation, and hygiene (WASH) model (Kang & Aldstadt, 2019). The Interagency Standing Committee (IASC) also promotes another model with a slightly different focus, specifically addressing "Disaster Risk Reduction and Climate Crises" (DRR)[27].

A key activity in the MHPSS model is educating and integrating the often insufficient number of medical and psychosocial professionals to respond effectively in humanitarian emergencies. Many MHPSS resources and materials are freely available on relevant websites [28], including the MHPSS Minimum Service Package. This package draws special attention to the rapid identification of service gaps and strategic, budget-conscious planning of effective interventions. Sharing models, resources, and experiences from past conflicts and disaster zones, along with tools like the accessible information movie clip "Meera and the Disaster Rewind Machine,"[29] enables adaptation and widespread use through open-access strategies online. This represents a significant opportunity for capacity building and facilitating broader dissemination and utilization of valuable resources.

It appears difficult to adequately evaluate the now widely accepted MHPSS interventions published online by the Interagency Standing Committee (IASC)[30] and Sphere[31].

Despite the obvious benefits, objective, independent evaluation and research of the MHPSS model and its components is developing slowly. This is likely due to the fact that the settings where the model is applied are complex and diverse and, therefore, difficult to compare. Nevertheless,

---

[26] See https://www.bmz.de/en/issues/displaced-people/mental-health-and-psychosocial-support-mhpss

[27] See https://www.ifrc.org/our-work/disasters-climate-and-crises

[28] See for example https://app.mhpss.net, accessed 14.1.2024

[29] Available from https://www.youtube.com/watch?v=FJOTrbOTS8I

[30] Inter-Agency Standing Committee (IASC) Reference Group for Mental Health and Psychosocial Support in Emergency Settings. A common monitoring and evaluation framework for mental health and psychosocial support in emergency settings. Geneva: IASC; 2017.

[31] https://app.mhpss.net/wp-content/uploads/2018/11/sphere-handbook-2018-en.pdf

some researchers from healthcare fields have taken up the challenge to independently appraise the guidelines or interventions in the MHPSS model (Duckers et al., 2022; Te Brake et al., 2022. For example, Duckers et al. (2022) reviewed and evaluated published MHPSS guidelines in the context of disaster risk reduction (DRR) (Te Brake et al., 2022). They identified "basic relief, information provision, emotional and social support, practical support, and health care" as the most common components in MHPSS guidelines. Their application of the Appraisal of Guidelines for Research and Evaluation-Health Systems (AGREE-HS) instrument indicated significant variation in the quality of the available guidelines. The authors concluded that MHPSS guidelines were "comprehensive, coherent, and sufficiently universal to serve as the "overarching framework"" (Duckers et al., 2022). Lasater et al. (2022) conducted a review of publications focusing on schools, children, and MHPSS. They identified 26 publications, reflecting 19 different published studies, in relevant databases. The authors found that there were different impacts of MHPSS in the context of schools/children depending on the different professionals involved, and user groups targeted. They recommended further research be done in this space. In 2014, O'Callaghan used case studies to list "lessons learned" in the application of MHPSS models with children (O'Callaghan, 2014). Riaz et al. (2023) recently proposed to make use of MHPSS models in other situations, like in areas affected by climate change-related natural disasters. Augustinavicius et al. (2018) also conducted a scoping review of 38 relevant MHPSS program documents and 89 relevant peer-reviewed articles. They drew attention to the lack of current evaluation standards and recommended steps to address this issue.

MHPSS models typically integrate ongoing monitoring and outcome evaluation strategies that might enhance quality assurance and allow for early correction of potential issues, supported by a recently published evaluation framework. Making this process public could benefit learning for similar situations and enable independent evaluations. However, publicizing these evaluations might complicate operations in already difficult circumstances. On the other hand, understanding the long-term impact and sustainability of outcomes should be addressed by more independent research, with both a health policy and interdisciplinary focus.

Internet-based and online services

Internet-based and online services have received increasing attention, especially since the global COVID-19 pandemic. These services include online counseling (Ierardi et al., 2022; Perin et al., 2023; Wilson et al., 2017) psychotherapy, diagnostic applications, telemedicine (Meng et al., 2020), social media-based interventions, and information systems. Research into the benefits of online, compared to in-person / on-site treatment, is still developing and requires further attention (Ierardi et al., 2022). In war or post-conflict areas, these types of online mental health services could be an essential strategy, especially in regions where geographical barriers and lack of infrastructure are a major barriers in service provision and health care training (Metz & Metz, 2022). Blended approaches might also be considered in these contexts (Meulenbroeks, 2020), and might be the best solution to combine the benefits of online and in-person models. Apps on smartphones have also been successfully tested for the delivery of therapies such as CBT. These services are even refunded in some health care systems, such as in Germany, and evaluation studies are ongoing. Midgeley et al. (2021) reported positive results in a pilot study which evaluated an Internet-Based Psychodynamic Treatment (iPDT) for Adolescents with Low Mood in the UK. The authors concluded that "preliminary data indicate that iPDT appears to be effective in reducing depressive symptoms in adolescents" (Midgley et al., 2021). Of course, essential prerequisites for these interventions include reliable, low-cost, or free internet services, as well as strategies to ensure data safety and confidentiality.

In the Iraq region that is the focus of the pilot project described in this book, the internet is generally accessible, even in many refugee camps. Internet-based approaches were therefore used in the project. The Internet also served the useful purpose of keeping contact between European partners and supervisors, students and teachers in the Iraq partner University, and NGOs benefitting from the project.

Concepts insufficiently covered by research: Collective and "group" trauma, second-generation and indirect trauma, and physical trauma with mental health symptoms

Groups, the search for meaning and collective trauma

While group or collective trauma (Kibel, 1973) are common terms in the literature, they are not covered in medical standard systems like the ICD and DSM. Medical research, therefore, tends to analyze epidemiological data on the prevalence of psychiatric disorders in violence-affected regions and communities, without considering possible differences between individuals and groups, and without following a comprehensive model that considers group or collective trauma. Psychodynamic concepts might be best for addressing this important aspect of mass violence.

Hirschberger (2018) recently analyzed the concept of group or collective trauma, and described the importance of loss of meaning: "Collective trauma is a cataclysmic event that shatters the basic fabric of society. Aside from the horrific loss of life, collective trauma is also a crisis of meaning". Somasundaram (2007, 2010), an experienced clinician, proposed a conceptualization of collective trauma using an interdisciplinary, multilevel, and socioeconomic approach. Several authors also link the problem to transgenerational transmission, which will be discussed separately in this chapter. Volkan has explored the difference between real group trauma and the feeling of historical group trauma. The latter can be created through political manipulation of groups by "bad leaders" to justify further violence (Volkan & Javakhishvili, 2022; Volkan, 2019, 2021). The concept of group or collective trauma is an ongoing discussion, which needs to be taken up in any region that has been exposed to mass violence.

Body to mind: Brain trauma and psychological symptoms resulting from physical illness

As described in our earlier sub-chapter on injuries in non-civilian populations, an insufficiently covered issue in both training and in research is blunt brain injuries, which are more common than generally considered. They are common in certain forms of violence, such as torture (Keatley et al., 2015; Mollica et al., 2014; Moreno & Grodin, 2002), war injuries, or exposure to explosions. They might be not detected when there is no obvious severe head injury, like fractures of the bone. Following instances of torture, abduction, and other forms of violence, survivors commonly report having experienced beatings to the head with different objects and being pushed against walls or to the floor. Exposure to blasts resulting from bombs or exploding ammunition can also lead to brain injuries (Quintana et al., 1997), even when no other injuries are obvious. A particular problem is that the post-concussive syndrome (PCS) symptoms resulting from these violent experiences can cover a broad range of problems, from headaches, dizziness, and vision impairment, to symptoms which are also common in PTSD. These symptoms range from irritability and sleep problems, to cognitive and memory problems, potentially reflecting changes in network connectivity (Nolan et al., 2021). These diagnoses are still predominantly based on clinical evaluations, as radio imaging strategies are often inconclusive. Special Nuclear Magnetic Imaging (NMR) can sometimes reveal subtle injuries (Sanchez-Carrion et al., 2008) such as small deposits of Hemosiderin (blood components) in some brain areas or axonal damage, but only when images follow specific protocols. Victims often become frustrated in treatment, especially if symptoms are treated as PTSD in psychotherapy, with no positive progress and potential worsening of symptoms. The potential benefits of treatment with Selective Serotonin Uptake Inhibitors (SSRI) medication for these patients is still controversial and under evaluation (Albrecht et al., 2018; Yue et al., 2017). Training with patients focusing on symptom improvement might be helpful if symptoms do not remit with time, but in post-conflict zones, experts with these special skills may be sparse or non-existent.

Chronic pain

Chronic pain is regularly observed after survivor's experience numerous possible war and violence-related physical injuries. For example, following land mine injuries, survivors may require amputations and experience phantom pain. In a study with Iranian war veterans, authors reported that after (transtibial) amputations patients reported "phantom sensations (54%), phantom pain (17%), stump pain (42%), but also lower back pain" (Ebrahimzadeh & Rajabi, 2007). In these cases, psychological and physical pain will interact and require competent, interdisciplinary treatment. Chronic pain which cannot be fully explained by physical findings, may also be a symptom of the cultural idiom of distress, especially when the expression of psychological symptoms is stigmatized. This should also be considered as an alternative explanation (Kohrt et al., 2021). In the context of "somatoform" pain disorders, especially when psychoanalytic concepts of conversion mechanisms are considered. Establishing resources for interdisciplinary treatment within university-based structures, as demonstrated in the Iraq pilot project, can be important for developing and providing training to professionals in this specialized field, integrating culturally sensitive psychotherapy.

Other somatic factors influencing or leading to psychological symptoms

It is important to consider that many physical illnesses, such as cardiac disease, diabetes, or even vitamin D deficiency resulting from malnutrition, can lead to or contribute to psychological symptoms like loss of energy, depression, or anxiety. All healthcare professionals working with patients in post-conflict settings, where it is common for patients to be overlooked and insufficiently treated, should be aware of this problem.

Again, a close interdisciplinary collaboration is essential for addressing this, and was implemented also in the project with the leading local teaching hospital. Successful psychotherapy may also improve the long-term outcomes of physical illnesses (Albus et al., 2011; Miller, 2002).

Cumulative trauma and trauma in children

Cumulative trauma is a concept which was first developed by Keilson (1980) to describe the impact of sequential traumatic events in children exposed to war or genocide. There are some conceptual differences regarding cumulative trauma in psychoanalytic and psychodynamic models, and in current standard medical terminology. The concept was explored in recent research by Finklestein and Solomon (2009) in Ethiopian refugee children. The research looked at trauma models offered by PTSD definitions and highlighted the importance of various experiences and psychosocial factors that require attention when considering refugee children (Finklestein & Solomon, 2009). Haselgruber et al. discussed issues with using the concepts of PTSD, complex PTSD, and disturbances in self-organization (DSO) (Kratzer et al., 2022). Further research may be required to better understand if these terms are merely different variations of the previously described Criterion A in the PTSD model. Resulting reactive disorders which are already defined in the DSM/ICD systems might require a new specific definition.

The concept of cumulative trauma may also need to be discussed in the context of the new models in ICD and DSM on childhood trauma. These models include attachment disorders, which often reflect sequential or cumulative trauma concepts and may also play a part in transgenerational transmission.

Attachment disorder (ICD 11)[32]

In the ICD-11, reactive attachment disorder is described as follows: "characterized by grossly abnormal attachment behaviors in early childhood, occurring in the context of a history of grossly inadequate childcare (e.g., severe neglect, maltreatment, institutional deprivation). Even when an adequate primary caregiver is newly available, the child does not turn to the primary caregiver for comfort, support, and nurture, rarely displays security-seeking behaviors towards any adult, and does not respond when

[32] See https://icd.who.int/browse/2024-01/mms/en#1867081699

comfort is offered. Reactive attachment disorder can only be diagnosed in children, and features of the disorder develop within the first 5 years of life. However, the disorder cannot be diagnosed before the age of 1 year (or a developmental age of less than 9 months), when the capacity for selective attachments may not be fully developed, or in the context of autism spectrum disorder."

The impact of trauma on children must be viewed as a specialized and important field, especially in war zones. A comprehensive overview of the impact of trauma on children in war zones is beyond the scope of this book.

Indirect victims and vicarious trauma

Given that violence is typically experienced by nearly all individuals in war areas, it is difficult to define "indirect" victims in post-conflict zones. Transgenerational trauma transmission can occur between individuals without direct exposure to experiences of violence, but rather through interactions with traumatized persons. This is one mechanism which helps us to understand that children and grandchildren of war victims may be considered indirect victims. In general, family members and others who are in close contact with victims can experience indirect traumatization. For example, a family member may have been a soldier (Ray & Vanstone, 2009), or might be a civilian who experienced traumatic events (Chartier-Otis et al., 2009). They may share their experiences verbally or nonverbally (Grunberg, 2022) with other family members, who may consequently develop symptoms of PTSD or other stress-related symptoms themselves. Survivors of direct violence may experience trauma spectrum disorders including PTSD or brain injury symptoms such as irritability, nightmares, and flashbacks. Victims may also experience difficulties with alcohol or substance abuse (Johnson et al., 2010) when they are used to cope with PTSD. Together, these symptoms and behaviors can lead to concern and distress, or other forms of psychological suffering in those close to the survivor.

Vicarious trauma: Therapists and helpers as indirect victims

Therapists or other helpers can develop "vicarious" trauma, including PTSD symptoms, or "compassion fatigue" through interactions with traumatized people during their professional work. Kizilhan has explored this problem with caregivers and mental health professionals in Iraq (Denkinger et al., 2018; Kizilhan, 2020), concluding that "better caring/support, supervision and organization are needed to enable psychotherapists to perform more effectively in war regions from the point of view of preventive healthcare." These recommendations were followed in the Duhok model project presented in this book. This requires sustainable and reliable support and self-care strategies for those working under difficult conditions and in direct contact with several traumatized victims. "Care-for-caregivers" strategies should be implemented as a key element in all teams working in war areas. This issue is often neglected and needs to receive more attention (Baker & Gabriel, 2021).

New "disorders"?

Several new categories have been included as psychological reactions or disorders which might be relevant and expected after violent conflicts. Examples of these new categories are presented in the next sub-section. Many of these new categories of mental health problems are still seen as preliminary and are part of ongoing discussions. These new mental health categories are not supported by an extensive body of research yet. In most cases, no established research instruments or questionnaires are available (at the time of writing this chapter), and especially not in validated form for different languages. Further, evidence-based treatment recommendations for these new mental health categories cannot be provided yet.

In cases like prolonged grief, it is important to give more consideration to cultural factors. The ways cultures express mourning and grief can vary significantly, affecting how these experiences are perceived and when they are considered pathological. Adapting definitions to be culturally sensitive may be required to avoid overly broad applications of these categories and their consequent treatments. In the next subsection, we present the most recent categories proposed by researchers or included as drafts in the recent DSM-5 and ICD revisions.

Prolonged grief disorder (PGD), bereavement, and sense of coherence

Prolonged grief disorder (PGD), also earlier described as "complicated" (29) or "pathological" grief, was added to the DSM-5 TR in 2022, after lengthy prior discussions (F 43.8). It was added to the same group as PTSD, and was also added in the ICD-11 (6B42) (Lenferink et al., 2021). Prolonged grief has always been acknowledged as a common reaction to loss and bereavement, though not always as a medical condition. It could be viewed as a trauma-specific or trauma-spectrum issue, as it typically involves a specific event with traumatic impact in the individuals' life. This is a common occurrence in many conflict and war regions. Several recent studies have started to explore different aspects and predictors of PGD, and questionnaires have been developed to measure the symptoms (Hyland et al., 2024). Research has explored the evidence-base for different interventions when addressing PGD. For example, Boelen et al. (2021) compared a CBT-based intervention with a supportive counseling intervention and found a better effect of CBT not only on PGD but also on PTSD and depression symptoms.

Sense of coherence (SOC), an important concept introduced by Antonovsky (REF), has been demonstrated to be relevant for recovery after traumatic events (Schafer et al. (2019)) SOC was also studied by Boelem and Connor (2022) as a factor in adjusting after bereavement. They assessed 221 Danish participants using the well-established SOC-29 and SOC-13 scales at 6, 13, and 18 months following a bereavement event. They found that meaningfulness was significant for adjustment, whereas manageability and comprehensibility were not as important in the SOC 12/29 model. The authors also highlighted a lack of a clearly defined self-image as a challenge in adjustment after bereavement (Boelen, 2012; Boelen et al., 2012).

In conflict zones and in similar settings, where supportive cultural structures and mourning rituals are disrupted or unavailable, adjustment to loss and bereavement might be especially difficult. We have observed this across different populations. In most cultures, solutions and supportive structures like burial rites and mourning periods are offered because death, loss, and bereavement may be viewed as common experiences in the cycle of life. Cultures and religion typically provide guidance and frameworks that support the coping process during these challenging times. Related to this, one of the most famous books in modern literature, James Joyce's seminal “Finnegans Wake”, can be interpreted as a reference to dreams (Cox, 1993) and the Irish tradition of a wake – a gathering to remember, share stories, and celebrate - after the death of a person. As recently as 1951, Patrick Leigh Fermor, a former intelligence operative, explored these concepts in the highly traditional Greek region of Mani (Fermor, 1958). He, and others, described various practices including complex death rituals. For example, years after death, relatives would compose and perform epic memorial poems to remember the achievements of the person who had passed[33]. In the context of mourning rituals, Pentaris (2012) writes about modern Greece: “If a woman does not wear black after the death of someone in the family, at least for one year, disrespect is shown to the deceased”. This illustrates that rituals can provide guidance and support, but also enforce social standards that sometimes might be hard to follow and create additional conflicts and distress. Death rituals may be seen as an obligation that needs to be fulfilled out of respect for religion, for the dead, or also to avoid restless and potentially dangerous spirits that might haunt the living. Most religions give concrete instructions on the obligations of the living, and especially of surviving family members, in these situations. In conflict and war areas, or areas under persecution, these different aspects of burial rites and mourning might be forcefully interrupted. When bodies or even body parts cannot be treated in the right way, and given the right farewell, normal processes of mourning and adjustment are disrupted. Consequently, conflict and suffering are to be expected in the survivors.

American authors, such as Kubler-Ross (1975), have proposed that a “regular” mourning process goes through several stages. This can typically be summarized as stages of “denial, anger, bargaining, depression, and acceptance.” However, it is unclear whether this model can be applied to all cultures and settings.

In mass atrocities in the context of modern warfare or major disasters like earthquakes, bodies often cannot be identified which interrupts normal rituals of mourning and coping, and cultural obligations to those who have died. Forensic projects aim to address this problem, using methods such as DNA testing and analyses of sources, to identify remains, reunite them with living relatives, and to provide closure. However, the dissemination of such findings can be delayed, potentially reaching relatives at different stages of the mourning process. This issue should be viewed as a psychological challenge, not just a technical or medical one (Carter, 1998; Stewart, 1999). This is crucial to consider in forensic projects, particularly in the identification and recovery of bodies.

Revenge and justice

At this point, we wish to further consider the importance of justice for mental health. In seeking justice for those killed, there can be a cultural expectation of revenge placed on survivors in many cultures, like Albania

[33] See for example Sokratis Kougeas: Τραγούδια του κάτω κόσμου. Μοιρολόγια της Μεσσηνιακής Μάνης. Το Ροδακιό Athens, 2000.

(Lopes Cardozo et al., 2003). This obligation is often seen as necessary to prevent conflicts that could hinder the adjustment to loss. Spirits of those slain not treated respectfully in death are already mentioned in the Ilias, when the slain Hector's spirit haunted Achilles, who had abused his body[34]. Achilles' reactions are also used as an example by some authors to explore the war trauma in Ukraine (Matiashova et al., 2022), with the respectful treatment of bodies and burials being a common problem in many war areas.

The correlation between feelings of a need for revenge and PTSD symptoms has recently been explored by several authors, mainly in soldiers, but also in victims of crime (Halimi et al., 2015; Muschalla et al., 2018; Neumann et al., 2021; van Denderen et al., 2014). The problem has also been observed in survivors of ISIS violence and was addressed in the project described in this book (Kizilhan & Neumann, 2020; Neumann et al., 2021). In various regions, initiatives involving transitional or restorative justice (Wenzel et al., 2021), and truth and reconciliation commissions, have addressed the issue of impunity among perpetrators. These efforts aim to promote societal recovery and to address mental health trauma in individual victims and groups (Cilliers et al., 2016; Stein, 1998; Stein et al., 1997; Swartz & Drennan, 2000). This approach was observed in post–NS Germany (Czech et al., 2023), before these models were fully developed.

Perpetrators

Perpetrators of violence are frequently overlooked in research. This is despite notable interviews with NS mass murderers published by Gilbert (1947) shortly after the Second World War. Other earlier work includes that by Haritas-Fatouros[35], who interviewed former torturers in Greece, and authors like Hanna Arendt (Sznaider, 2011), who underlined that many perpetrators were not perverted exotic monsters, but apparently friendly and "normal" persons, or even neighbors of their later victims.

More recently, research has explored religious (Mirzaei et al., 2011) and other "absolute" belief systems which can be used to select and manipulate vulnerable target groups to become perpetrators (Kizilhan & Cavelius, 2016). The group analyst Vamik Volkan (1980, 1987, 2021) has

---

[34] *Iliad* Book XXIV, ll. 18-23

[35] See https://academic.oup.com/bjc/article-abstract/43/4/817/348526?redirectedFrom=fulltext&login=false

described manipulation of groups by "bad leaders" in the lead-up to genocide and mass violence, as noted before. This is done using the concepts of "Chosen" (group) traumas and glories, which are used to create group identities based on fictitious historical concepts.

Stigma

In many cultures, mental health is severely stigmatized. Even in Europe and the US, changes in public perceptions are relatively slow. This is an issue for patients but also for mental health services, their institutions, service providers, and healthcare professionals (Dow & Siniscarco, 2021; Molloy et al., 2020). Young medical professionals may avoid becoming psychiatrists, which might contribute to the low availability of necessary professionals and services, especially in disaster and war situations. Several experts and organizations have taken proactive steps, especially through social and online media platforms, to reduce stigma associated with mental health issues. Movies starring famous actors speaking openly about mental health issues, as role models, could potentially be helpful in reducing stigma and improving health literacy in the general public (Sabin et al., 2022). This approach parallels efforts seen in reporting on suicide (Fu & Yip, 2008), though stigma may persist during direct contact with patients and their family members. Stigma surrounding mental health might stem from several factors: fear of hereditary implications, historical practices like detaining patients under adverse conditions or even subjecting them to torture and killing - especially in the NS era - and historically limited treatment options which continue to economically burden caregivers. Insurance systems may also exacerbate this issue by avoiding the costs associated with mental health care, again due to stigma.

The stigma associated with mental health may explain the preference for patients to focus on physical symptoms. This preference contributes to the "somatization" discussion in transcultural medicine, where psychological distress is expressed through physical symptoms. This stigma creates barriers to treatment seeking and influences health belief models, causing people to avoid addressing stigmatized mental health issues (Raguram & Weiss, 2004; Raguram et al., 1996). Exploring health belief models which lead to stigma, generally through qualitative research first, might be necessary for preparing interventions and addressing cultural illness formulations that might play a role in a given context.

Anti-stigma campaigns were included in the pilot project presented in this book. These campaigns utilized various approaches, including social media, brochures, training programs for multipliers, and changes in the portrayal of mental health issues in movies (Hankir et al., 2017; Quinn et al., 2011; Zheng et al., 2016). These efforts, supported by governments and various respected social groups, emphasized the collective responsibility of all members of society to bring about change. The World Psychiatric Association (WPA) has started a major Anti-Stigma campaign in this context[36], and special campaigns for conditions such as Schizophrenia[37]. Anti-stigma campaigns specifically addressing trauma spectrum disorders are still mainly targeted towards soldiers and veterans (Blais & Renshaw, 2013; Hooyer, 2022; Phelan et al., 2011), but should be extended to also include civilian victims. The effectiveness of anti-stigma interventions, particularly in the long-term, depends on cultural context. Therefore, a careful early assessment of the specific cultural and social factors is crucial. This assessment could help guide the strategy and selection of appropriate tools, to ensure they align with the identified factors in a given environment. In some settings, low-technology media like radio might be the most realistic option, as radios can be operated with solar energy and without Internet. However, TV and internet-based media are increasingly capturing communities' attention, even in many refugee camps, such as the long-term camps in northern Iraq featured in our project. In the absence of accurate information being provided by reliable experts, rumors, false information, and health belief models can mislead large groups of individuals, especially in the presence of rapidly developing internet-based media (Southwell et al., 2019). Media health literacy (MHL) has been identified as a new concern in this context (Parandeh Afshar et al., 2022; Zuair & Sopory, 2022).

In this context, the strategies used in anti-stigma campaigns can likely be applied to related areas, such as building general health literacy, raising awareness, and influencing health belief models. However, as previously noted, it is crucial to conduct a thorough assessment of cultural, economic, and technical conditions in advance, to avoid wasting resources, corruption, and inefficient strategies. A well-planned media strategy is expected to be a key element in improving the situation for patients and health care services. Therefore, media experts already working within the regions may be essential members of interdisciplinary teams, who could also benefit from training and capacity building in this area.

---

[36] https://www.wpanet.org/stigma-and-mental-illness

[37] Sartorius N, Schulze H, Reducing the stigma of mental illness. A report from a global program of the World Psychiatric Association. Cambridge University Press, Cambridge, 2005

To summarize: In addition to in-person educational and informational meetings, internet-based interventions that promote critical health literacy and provide reliable health information and resources should be considered in strategic planning. These can be combined with efforts to improve internet access or distribute printed media when necessary. Interventions and resources should be culturally-sensitive and in local languages, with available tools adapted to fit these requirements. Integrating prominent individuals from communities, such as actors or religious authorities, might contribute to the acceptance of interventions/campaigns. As with all activities, commitments should be made based on the resources that are actually available. If treatment and services that are then not freely available or accessible are promoted in a campaign, it might backfire and create new problems. Sustainability is again a key priority in this context, and long-term external funding might be necessary to maintain efforts to raise awareness, and to support long-term service provision in a balanced way. This is especially important given chronic problems will often require long-term treatment and support.

It should be noted again that the WHO and other international organizations are already offering free tools in many areas, including mental health support for the general public. The WHO has published a website containing relevant including media-related tools[38].

References

Agaibi, C. E., & Wilson, J. P. (2005, Jul). Trauma, PTSD, and resilience: a review of the literature. *Trauma Violence Abuse, 6*(3), 195-216. https://doi.org/10.1177/1524838005277438

Aggarwal, N. K. (2023, Jun). The Evolving Culture Concept in Psychiatric Cultural Formulation: Implications for Anthropological Theory and Psychiatric Practice. *Cult Med Psychiatry, 47*(2), 555-575. https://doi.org/10.1007/s11013-023-09821-9

Aggarwal, N. K., Chen, D., & Lewis-Fernandez, R. (2023). Eliciting social stressors, supports, and determinants of health through the DSM-5 cultural formulation interview. *Front Psychiatry, 14*, 1148170. https://doi.org/10.3389/fpsyt.2023.1148170

Al Shawi, A. F., & Hassen, S. M. (2022, May). Traumatic events, post-traumatic stress disorders, and gender among Yazidi population after

[38] See https://www.who.int/tools

ISIS invasion: A post conflict study in Kurdistan - Iraq. *Int J Soc Psychiatry, 68*(3), 656-661. https://doi.org/10.1177/0020764021994145

Albrecht, J. S., Rao, V., Perfetto, E. M., & Daniel Mullins, C. (2018, Aug). Safety of Antidepressant Classes Used Following Traumatic Brain Injury Among Medicare Beneficiaries: A Retrospective Cohort Study. *Drugs Aging, 35*(8), 763-772. https://doi.org/10.1007/s40266-018-0570-2

Albus, C., Beutel, M. E., Deter, H. C., Fritzsche, K., Hellmich, M., Jordan, J., Juenger, J., Krauth, C., Ladwig, K. H., Michal, M., Mueck-Weymann, M., Petrowski, K., Pieske, B., Ronel, J., Soellner, W., Waller, C., Weber, C., & Herrmann-Lingen, C. (2011, Oct). A stepwise psychotherapy intervention for reducing risk in coronary artery disease (SPIRR-CAD) - rationale and design of a multicenter, randomized trial in depressed patients with CAD. *J Psychosom Res, 71*(4), 215-222. https://doi.org/10.1016/j.jpsychores.2011.02.013

Amone-P'Olak, K., Stochl, J., Ovuga, E., Abbott, R., Meiser-Stedman, R., Croudace, T. J., & Jones, P. B. (2014, May). Postwar environment and long-term mental health problems in former child soldiers in Northern Uganda: the WAYS study. *J Epidemiol Community Health, 68*(5), 425-430. https://doi.org/10.1136/jech-2013-203042

Anderson, C., & McCarley, M. (2013, May-Jun). Psychological birth trauma in adolescents experiencing an early birth. *MCN Am J Matern Child Nurs, 38*(3), 170-176. https://doi.org/10.1097/NMC.0b013e31826f6cad

Antonovsky, A. (2022). Salutogenesis and Mental Health Promotion in Military Settings. In M. B. Mittelmark, G. F. Bauer, L. Vaandrager, J. M. Pelikan, S. Sagy, M. Eriksson, B. Lindstrom, & C. Meier Magistretti (Eds.), *The Handbook of Salutogenesis* (2nd ed., pp. 337-348). https://doi.org/10.1007/978-3-030-79515-3_32

Augustinavicius, J. L., Greene, M. C., Lakin, D. P., & Tol, W. A. (2018). Monitoring and evaluation of mental health and psychosocial support programs in humanitarian settings: a scoping review of terminology and focus. *Confl Health, 12*, 9. https://doi.org/10.1186/s13031-018-0146-0

Baker, C., & Gabriel, L. (2021, 2021/05/04). Exploring how therapists engage in self-care in times of personal distress. *British Journal of Guidance & Counselling, 49*(3), 435-444. https://doi.org/10.1080/03069885.2021.1885010

Baldwin, D. V. (2013, Sep). Primitive mechanisms of trauma response: an evolutionary perspective on trauma-related disorders. *Neurosci Biobehav Rev, 37*(8), 1549-1566.

https://doi.org/10.1016/j.neubiorev.2013.06.004

Barrash, J., Denburg, N. L., Moser, D. J., Woolson, R. F., Schumacher, A. J., & Doebbeling, B. N. (2007, Jul). Credibility of neuropsychological performances of Persian Gulf War veterans and military control subjects participating in clinical epidemiological research. *Mil Med, 172*(7), 697-707. https://doi.org/10.7205/milmed.172.7.697

Basoglu, M. (2009, Apr). A multivariate contextual analysis of torture and cruel, inhuman, and degrading treatments: implications for an evidence-based definition of torture. *Am J Orthopsychiatry, 79*(2), 135-145. https://doi.org/10.1037/a0015681

Beckmann, J., Wenzel, T., Hautzinger, M., & Kizilhan, J. I. (2022). Training of psychotherapists in post-conflict regions: A Community case study in the Kurdistan Region of Iraq. *Front Psychiatry, 13*, 947903. https://doi.org/10.3389/fpsyt.2022.947903

Berthold, S. M., Mollica, R. F., Silove, D., Tay, A. K., Lavelle, J., & Lindert, J. (2019, Jun 1). The HTQ-5: revision of the Harvard Trauma Questionnaire for measuring torture, trauma and DSM-5 PTSD symptoms in refugee populations. *Eur J Public Health, 29*(3), 468-474. https://doi.org/10.1093/eurpub/cky256

Betancourt, T. S. (2008, Apr). Child soldiers: reintegration, pathways to recovery, and reflections from the field. *J Dev Behav Pediatr, 29*(2), 138-141. https://doi.org/10.1097/DBP.0b013e31816be946

Betancourt, T. S. (2010, Jul). A Longitudinal Study of Psychosocial Adjustment and Community Reintegration among Former Child Soldiers in Sierra Leone. *Int Psychiatry, 7*(3), 60-62. https://doi.org/10.1192/s1749367600005853

Betancourt, T. S., Borisova, II, Williams, T. P., Brennan, R. T., Whitfield, T. H., de la Soudiere, M., Williamson, J., & Gilman, S. E. (2010, Jul-Aug). Sierra Leone's former child soldiers: a follow-up study of psychosocial adjustment and community reintegration. *Child Dev, 81*(4), 1077-1095. https://doi.org/10.1111/j.1467-8624.2010.01455.x

Betancourt, T. S., Borisova, I., Williams, T. P., Meyers-Ohki, S. E., Rubin-Smith, J. E., Annan, J., & Kohrt, B. A. (2013, Jan). Psychosocial adjustment and mental health in former child soldiers--systematic review of the literature and recommendations for future research. *J Child Psychol Psychiatry, 54*(1), 17-36. https://doi.org/10.1111/j.1469-7610.2012.02620.x

Betancourt, T. S., Simmons, S., Borisova, I., Brewer, S. E., Iweala, U., & Soudiere, M. D. (2008, Nov 1). High Hopes, Grim Reality: Reintegration and the Education of Former Child Soldiers in Sierra Leone. *Comp Educ Rev, 52*(4), 565-587. https://doi.org/10.1086/591298

Blais, R. K., & Renshaw, K. D. (2013, Feb). Stigma and demographic correlates of help-seeking intentions in returning service members. *J Trauma Stress, 26*(1), 77-85. https://doi.org/10.1002/jts.21772

Boelen, P. A. (2012, Mar). A prospective examination of the association between the centrality of a loss and post-loss psychopathology. *J Affect Disord, 137*(1-3), 117-124. https://doi.org/10.1016/j.jad.2011.12.004

Boelen, P. A., Keijsers, L., & van den Hout, M. A. (2012, Jan). The role of self-concept clarity in prolonged grief disorder. *J Nerv Ment Dis, 200*(1), 56-62. https://doi.org/10.1097/NMD.0b013e31823e577f

Boelen, P. A., Lenferink, L. I. M., & Spuij, M. (2021, Apr 1). CBT for Prolonged Grief in Children and Adolescents: A Randomized Clinical Trial. *Am J Psychiatry, 178*(4), 294-304. https://doi.org/10.1176/appi.ajp.2020.20050548

Boelen, P. A., & O'Connor, M. (2022, Sep). Is a sense of coherence associated with prolonged grief, depression, and satisfaction with life after bereavement? A longitudinal study. *Clin Psychol Psychother, 29*(5), 1599-1610. https://doi.org/10.1002/cpp.2774

Borisova, L. V., Martinussen, P. E., Rydland, H. T., Stornes, P., & Eikemo, T. A. (2017, Mar). Public evaluation of health services across 21 European countries: The role of culture. *Scand J Public Health, 45*(2), 132-139. https://doi.org/10.1177/1403494816685920

Brewin, C. R., Andrews, B., Rose, S., & Kirk, M. (1999, Mar). Acute stress disorder and posttraumatic stress disorder in victims of violent crime. *Am J Psychiatry, 156*(3), 360-366. https://doi.org/10.1176/ajp.156.3.360

Bruenig, D., Mehta, D., Morris, C. P., Lawford, B., Harvey, W., Mc, D. Y. R., & Voisey, J. (2018, Feb). Correlation between interferon gamma and interleukin 6 with PTSD and resilience. *Psychiatry Res, 260*, 193-198. https://doi.org/10.1016/j.psychres.2017.11.069

Cantor, C. (2009, Nov). Post-traumatic stress disorder: evolutionary perspectives. *Aust N Z J Psychiatry, 43*(11), 1038-1048. https://doi.org/10.3109/00048670903270407

Carter, Y. H. (1998, Nov). Death notification and bereavement in general practice: optimizing the quality of care. *Br J Gen Pract, 48*(436), 1728-1729. https://www.ncbi.nlm.nih.gov/pubmed/10198477

Casey, P. (2014, Jun). Adjustment disorder: new developments. *Curr Psychiatry Rep, 16*(6), 451. https://doi.org/10.1007/s11920-014-0451-2

Chartier-Otis, M., Guay, S., & Marchand, A. (2009, Jul). Psychological and relationship distress among partners of civilian PTSD patients. *J Nerv Ment Dis, 197*(7), 543-546. https://doi.org/10.1097/NMD.0b013e3181aac807

Cilliers, J., Dube, O., & Siddiqi, B. (2016, May 13). Reconciling after civil conflict increases social capital but decreases individual well-being. *Science, 352*(6287), 787-794. https://doi.org/10.1126/science.aad9682

Colamaria, A., Blagia, M., Carbone, F., & Fochi, N. P. (2022). Blast-related traumatic brain injury: Report of a severe case and review of the literature. *Surg Neurol Int, 13*, 151. https://doi.org/10.25259/SNI_1134_2021

Committee on Public, E. (2000, Jul-Sep). Committee on Publication Ethics (COPE). Guidelines on good publication practice. *J Postgrad Med, 46*(3), 217-221. https://www.ncbi.nlm.nih.gov/pubmed/11298477

Correa-Chica, A., Caicedo-Moreno, A., Rincon-Unigarro, C., Castro-Abril, P., & Lopez-Lopez, W. (2024, Jun). Episodic versus thematic media framing of violence against social leaders and human rights defenders in Colombia. *Int J Psychol, 59*(3), 390-397. https://doi.org/10.1002/ijop.13113

Cox, O. (1993, Aug). Some dream mechanisms in Finnegans Wake. *Int J Psychoanal, 74 (Pt 4)*, 815-821. https://www.ncbi.nlm.nih.gov/pubmed/8407134

Crocq, M. A., & Crocq, L. (2000, Mar). From shell shock and war neurosis to posttraumatic stress disorder: a history of psychotraumatology. *Dialogues Clin Neurosci, 2*(1), 47-55. https://doi.org/10.31887/DCNS.2000.2.1/macrocq

Cukor, J., Olden, M., Lee, F., & Difede, J. (2010, Oct). Evidence-based treatments for PTSD, new directions, and special challenges. *Ann N Y Acad Sci, 1208*, 82-89. https://doi.org/10.1111/j.1749-6632.2010.05793.x

Czech, H., Hildebrandt, S., Reis, S. P., Chelouche, T., Fox, M., Gonzalez-Lopez, E., Lepicard, E., Ley, A., Offer, M., Ohry, A., Rotzoll, M., Sachse, C., Siegel, S. J., Simunek, M., Teicher, A., Uzarczyk, K., von Villiez, A., Wald, H. S., Wynia, M. K., & Roelcke, V. (2023, Nov 18). The Lancet Commission on medicine, Nazism, and the Holocaust: historical evidence, implications for today, teaching for tomorrow. *Lancet, 402*(10415), 1867-1940. https://doi.org/10.1016/S0140-6736(23)01845-7

Dayan, J., & Olliac, B. (2010, Dec). From hysteria and shell shock to posttraumatic stress disorder: comments on psychoanalytic and neuropsychological approaches. *J Physiol Paris, 104*(6), 296-302. https://doi.org/10.1016/j.jphysparis.2010.09.003

Denkinger, J. K., Windthorst, P., Rometsch-Ogioun El Sount, C., Blume, M., Sedik, H., Kizilhan, J. I., Gibbons, N., Pham, P., Hillebrecht, J., Ateia, N., Nikendei, C., Zipfel, S., & Junne, F. (2018). Secondary Traumatization in Caregivers Working With Women and Children

Who Suffered Extreme Violence by the "Islamic State". *Front Psychiatry, 9*, 234. https://doi.org/10.3389/fpsyt.2018.00234

Dow, C., & Siniscarco, M. (2021, Feb 1). Culture, Mental Health, and Stigma. *J Psychosoc Nurs Ment Health Serv, 59*(2), 5. https://doi.org/10.3928/02793695-20210114-02

Duckers, M., van Hoof, W., Willems, A., & Te Brake, H. (2022, Jun 25). Appraising Evidence-Based Mental Health and Psychosocial Support (MHPSS) Guidelines-PART II: A Content Analysis with Implications for Disaster Risk Reduction. *Int J Environ Res Public Health, 19*(13). https://doi.org/10.3390/ijerph19137798

Ebrahimzadeh, M. H., & Rajabi, M. T. (2007, Nov-Dec). Long-term outcomes of patients undergoing war-related amputations of the foot and ankle. *J Foot Ankle Surg, 46*(6), 429-433. https://doi.org/10.1053/j.jfas.2007.08.011

Eitinger, L. (1961, Oct). Pathology of the concentration camp syndrome. Preliminary report. *Arch Gen Psychiatry, 5*, 371-379. https://doi.org/10.1001/archpsyc.1961.01710160051006

Eitinger, L. (1962, Apr). Concentration camp survivors in the postwar world. *Am J Orthopsychiatry, 32*, 367-375. https://doi.org/10.1111/j.1939-0025.1962.tb00283.x

Elhai, J. D., Franklin, C. L., & Gray, M. J. (2008). The SCID PTSD module's trauma screen: validity with two samples in detecting trauma history. *Depress Anxiety, 25*(9), 737-741. https://doi.org/10.1002/da.20318

Engel, C. C., Jr. (2004, Summer). Post-war syndromes: illustrating the impact of the social psyche on notions of risk, responsibility, reason, and remedy. *J Am Acad Psychoanal Dyn Psychiatry, 32*(2), 321-334; discussion 335-343. https://doi.org/10.1521/jaap.32.2.321.35275

Ernst, E. (1996, May). Killing in the name of healing: the active role of the German medical profession during the Third Reich. *Am J Med, 100*(5), 579-581. https://doi.org/10.1016/s0002-9343(96)00006-x

Ernst, E. (1997). 50 years ago: the Nuremberg Doctors' Tribunal. Part 4: Nazi medicine's relevance today. *Wien Med Wochenschr, 147*(3), 70-71. https://www.ncbi.nlm.nih.gov/pubmed/9086587

Fabra, M. (2003, Mar 1). [The so-called trauma criterium (A--Criterium in DSM-IV) of post-traumatic stress disorder and its significance for social and legal insurance (II)]. *Versicherungsmedizin, 55*(1), 19-26. https://www.ncbi.nlm.nih.gov/pubmed/12652928 (Das sogenannte Traumakriterium (A-Kriterium des DSM-IV) der Posttraumatischen Belastungsstorung und seine Bedeutung fur die Sozial- und Sachversicherung (II).)

Fares, Y., Fares, J., & Gebeily, S. (2014, Jun). Head and facial injuries due to cluster munitions. *Neurol Sci, 35*(6), 905-910. https://doi.org/10.1007/s10072-013-1623-2

Fermor, P. L. (1958). *Mani; travels in the southern Peloponnese*. Harper.

Finklestein, M., & Solomon, Z. (2009). Cumulative trauma, PTSD and dissociation among Ethiopian refugees in Israel. *J Trauma Dissociation, 10*(1), 38-56. https://doi.org/10.1080/15299730802485151

Fischer-Homberger, E. (1970). [Railway spine and traumatic neuroses--the psyche and the spinal cord]. *Gesnerus, 27*(1-2), 96-111. https://www.ncbi.nlm.nih.gov/pubmed/4928375 (Railway Spine und traumatische Neurose--Steele und Ruckenmark.)

Fu, K. W., & Yip, P. S. (2008, Oct). Changes in reporting of suicide news after the promotion of the WHO media recommendations. *Suicide Life Threat Behav, 38*(5), 631-636. https://doi.org/10.1521/suli.2008.38.5.631

Gilbert, G. M. (1947). *Nuremberg diary*. Farrar, Straus.

Gold, L. H. (1998). Addressing bias in the forensic assessment of sexual harassment claims. *J Am Acad Psychiatry Law, 26*(4), 563-578. https://www.ncbi.nlm.nih.gov/pubmed/9894213

Grunberg, K. (2022, Sep). Afterwards-Forgetting, Remembering, Transmitting. Extreme Trauma and Culture in Post-National-Socialist Germany. *Am J Psychoanal, 82*(3), 405-425. https://doi.org/10.1057/s11231-022-09368-5

Gutierrez-Pelaez, M., & Herrera-Pardo, E. (2017, Apr-Jun). [Environment, Trauma and Technical Innovations: Three Links Between Donald W. Winnicott and Sandor Ferenczi]. *Rev Colomb Psiquiatr, 46*(2), 121-126. https://doi.org/10.1016/j.rcp.2015.12.001 (Ambiente, trauma e innovaciones tecnicas: tres articulaciones entre Donald W. Winnicott y Sandor Ferenczi.)

Hagan, J., & Kaiser, J. (2011, Mar). The displaced and dispossessed of Darfur: explaining the sources of a continuing state-led genocide. *Br J Sociol, 62*(1), 1-25. https://doi.org/10.1111/j.1468-4446.2011.01357.x

Halimi, R., Dragoti, E., Halimi, H., Sylejmani-Hulaj, N., & Jashari-Ramadani, S. (2015, Feb 24). Socio-Cultural Context and Feelings of Hatred and Revenge in War Veterans with Post-Traumatic Stress Disorder 15 Years after War in Kosovo. *Ment Illn, 7*(1), 5609. https://doi.org/10.4081/mi.2015.5609

Hankir, A., Zaman, R., Geers, B., Rosie, G., Breslin, G., Barr, L., Carrick, F. R., & Anderson, S. (2017, Sep). The Wounded Healer film: A London College of Communication event to challenge mental health stigma through the power of motion picture. *Psychiatr Danub, 29*(Suppl 3), 307-312. https://www.ncbi.nlm.nih.gov/pubmed/28953783

Hankoff, L. D. (1988). The Illness Narrative: Suffering, Healing, and the Human Condition. *JAMA, 260*(6), 859-860. https://doi.org/10.1001/jama.1988.03410060135047

Harrington, R. (1996, Jan). The "railway spine" diagnosis and Victorian responses to PTSD. *J Psychosom Res, 40*(1), 11-14. https://doi.org/10.1016/0022-3999(95)00514-5

Hausotter, W. (1996, Aug 1). [Expert assessment of railroad accidents at the beginning of the industrial age--a medical historical excursion with reference to current circumstances]. *Versicherungsmedizin, 48*(4), 138-142. https://www.ncbi.nlm.nih.gov/pubmed/8966852 (Die Begutachtung der Eisenbahnunfalle am Beginn des Industriezeitalters--Ein medizinhistorischer Exkurs mit Bezug zur Gegenwart.)

Heisler, M., Lin, J., Modvig, J., Esdaile, C., & Iacopino, V. (2022, Nov 26). Free Sebnem Korur Fincanci and end systematic silencing of health professionals. *Lancet, 400*(10366), 1843-1844. https://doi.org/10.1016/S0140-6736(22)02359-5

Hensel-Dittmann, D., Schauer, M., Ruf, M., Catani, C., Odenwald, M., Elbert, T., & Neuner, F. (2011). Treatment of traumatized victims of war and torture: a randomized controlled comparison of narrative exposure therapy and stress inoculation training. *Psychother Psychosom, 80*(6), 345-352. https://doi.org/10.1159/000327253

Hirschberger, G. (2018). Collective Trauma and the Social Construction of Meaning. *Front Psychol, 9*, 1441. https://doi.org/10.3389/fpsyg.2018.01441

Hooyer, K. (2022). The "trauma pitch": How stigma emerges for Iraq and Afghanistan veterans seeking disability compensation. *PLoS One, 17*(8), e0267424. https://doi.org/10.1371/journal.pone.0267424

Humphreys, G. (2009, May). Healing child soldiers. *Bull World Health Organ, 87*(5), 330-331. https://doi.org/10.2471/blt.09.020509

Hyland, P., Hamer, R., Fox, R., Vallieres, F., Karatzias, T., Shevlin, M., & Cloitre, M. (2024, Jan-Feb). Is Dissociation a Fundamental Component of ICD-11 Complex Posttraumatic Stress Disorder? *J Trauma Dissociation, 25*(1), 45-61. https://doi.org/10.1080/15299732.2023.2231928

Iacopino, V., Haar, R. J., Heisler, M., Lin, J., Fincanci, S. K., Esdaile, C., Modvig, J., Sveaass, N., Nathanson, V. H., Melzer, N., & Cohen, J. (2022, Jul 16). Istanbul Protocol 2022 empowers health professionals to end torture. *Lancet, 400*(10347), 143-145. https://doi.org/10.1016/S0140-6736(22)00948-5

Ibrahim, H., Ertl, V., Catani, C., Ismail, A. A., & Neuner, F. (2018, Sep 13). Trauma and perceived social rejection among Yazidi women and girls who survived enslavement and genocide. *BMC Med, 16*(1), 154. https://doi.org/10.1186/s12916-018-1140-5

Ierardi, E., Bottini, M., & Riva Crugnola, C. (2022, Feb 22). Effectiveness of an online versus face-to-face psychodynamic counselling intervention for university students before and during the COVID-19 period. *BMC Psychol, 10*(1), 35. https://doi.org/10.1186/s40359-022-00742-7

International Council on Human Rights Policy. (1999). *Hard cases : bringing human rights violators to justice abroad : a guide to universal jurisdiction*. International Council on Human Rights Policy.

Johnson, S. D., Cottler, L. B., O'Leary, C. C., & Ben Abdallah, A. (2010, Nov-Dec). The association of trauma and PTSD with the substance use profiles of alcohol- and cocaine-dependent out-of-treatment women. *Am J Addict, 19*(6), 490-495. https://doi.org/10.1111/j.1521-0391.2010.00075.x

Jones, E. (2006, Apr 29). Historical approaches to post-combat disorders. *Philos Trans R Soc Lond B Biol Sci, 361*(1468), 533-542. https://doi.org/10.1098/rstb.2006.1814

Jorgensen, U., Melchiorsen, H., Gottlieb, A. G., Hallas, V., & Nielsen, C. V. (2010). Using the International Classification of Functioning, Disability and Health (ICF) to describe the functioning of traumatised refugees. *Torture, 20*(2), 57-75.
https://www.ncbi.nlm.nih.gov/pubmed/20952823

Kabengele Mpinga, E., & Chastonay, P. (2005, Sep). [Health and human rights: perceptions of health professionals and human rights defenders]. *Sante Publique, 17*(3), 371-383.
https://doi.org/10.3917/spub.053.0371 (Sante et droits humains: perceptions de leurs defenseurs et des professionnels de sante.)

Kang, J. Y., & Aldstadt, J. (2019, Aug). Examining time-dependent effects of water, sanitation, and hygiene (WASH) interventions using an agent-based model. *Trop Med Int Health, 24*(8), 962-971. https://doi.org/10.1111/tmi.13280

Keatley, E., d'Alfonso, A., Abeare, C., Keller, A., & Bertelsen, N. S. (2015, Nov-Dec). Health Outcomes of Traumatic Brain Injury Among Refugee Survivors of Torture. *J Head Trauma Rehabil, 30*(6), E1-8. https://doi.org/10.1097/HTR.0000000000000103

Keilson, H. (1980, Nov). Sequential traumatization of children. *Dan Med Bull, 27*(5), 235-237. https://www.ncbi.nlm.nih.gov/pubmed/7449450

Keshavan, M. S. (2014, Dec). Culture bound syndromes: disease entities or simply concepts of distress? *Asian J Psychiatr, 12*, 1-2. https://doi.org/10.1016/j.ajp.2014.11.003

Kibel, H. D. (1973, Jan). A group member's suicide: treating collective trauma. *Int J Group Psychother, 23*(1), 42-53. https://doi.org/10.1080/00207284.1973.11492208

Kim, Y. (2012). [Historical perspective of PTSD and future revision in DSM-5]. *Seishin Shinkeigaku Zasshi, 114*(9), 1031-1036. https://www.ncbi.nlm.nih.gov/pubmed/23198592

Kizilhan, I., & Cavelius, A. (2016). *Die Psychologie des IS : die Logik der Massenmörder*. Europa Verlag.

Kizilhan, J. I. (2014, Jun). Religious and cultural aspects of psychotherapy in Muslim patients from tradition-oriented societies. *Int Rev Psychiatry, 26*(3), 335-343. https://doi.org/10.3109/09540261.2014.899203

Kizilhan, J. I. (2020, Mar 10). Stress on local and international psychotherapists in the crisis region of Iraq. *BMC Psychiatry, 20*(1), 110. https://doi.org/10.1186/s12888-020-02508-0

Kizilhan, J. I., Berger, T., Sennhauser, L., & Wenzel, T. (2023). The psychological impact of genocide on the Yazidis. *Front Psychol, 14*, 1074283. https://doi.org/10.3389/fpsyg.2023.1074283

Kizilhan, J. I., Friedl, N., Neumann, J., & Traub, L. (2020, May 24). Potential trauma events and the psychological consequences for Yazidi women after ISIS captivity. *BMC Psychiatry, 20*(1), 256. https://doi.org/10.1186/s12888-020-02671-4

Kizilhan, J. I., & Neumann, J. (2020). The Significance of Justice in the Psychotherapeutic Treatment of Traumatized People After War and Crises. *Front Psychiatry, 11*, 540. https://doi.org/10.3389/fpsyt.2020.00540

Kizilhan, J. I., & Noll-Hussong, M. (2018, Jul). Post-traumatic stress disorder among former Islamic State child soldiers in northern Iraq. *Br J Psychiatry, 213*(1), 425-429. https://doi.org/10.1192/bjp.2018.88

Kizilhan, J. I., Noll-Hussong, M., & Wenzel, T. (2021, Dec 22). Transgenerational Transmission of Trauma across Three Generations of Alevi Kurds. *Int J Environ Res Public Health, 19*(1). https://doi.org/10.3390/ijerph19010081

Kizilhan, J. I., Steger, F., & Noll-Hussong, M. (2020, Mar). Shame, dissociative seizures and their correlation among traumatised female Yazidi with experience of sexual violence. *Br J Psychiatry, 216*(3), 138-143. https://doi.org/10.1192/bjp.2020.2

Kizilhan, J. I., & Wenzel, T. (2020, Nov-Dec). Positive psychotherapy in the treatment of traumatised Yezidi survivors of sexualised violence and genocide. *Int Rev Psychiatry, 32*(7-8), 594-605.

https://doi.org/10.1080/09540261.2020.1809356

Klasen, F., Oettingen, G., Daniels, J., & Adam, H. (2010, Oct). Multiple trauma and mental health in former Ugandan child soldiers. *J Trauma Stress, 23*(5), 573-581. https://doi.org/10.1002/jts.20557

Klasen, F., Oettingen, G., Daniels, J., Post, M., Hoyer, C., & Adam, H. (2010, Jul-Aug). Posttraumatic resilience in former Ugandan child soldiers. *Child Dev, 81*(4), 1096-1113. https://doi.org/10.1111/j.1467-8624.2010.01456.x

Klasen, F., Reissmann, S., Voss, C., & Okello, J. (2015, Apr). The guiltless guilty: trauma-related guilt and psychopathology in former Ugandan child soldiers. *Child Psychiatry Hum Dev, 46*(2), 180-193. https://doi.org/10.1007/s10578-014-0470-6

Kohrt, B. A., Jordans, M. J. D., Turner, E. L., Rai, S., Gurung, D., Dhakal, M., Bhardwaj, A., Lamichhane, J., Singla, D. R., Lund, C., Patel, V., Luitel, N. P., & Sikkema, K. J. (2021, Nov 1). Collaboration With People With Lived Experience of Mental Illness to Reduce Stigma and Improve Primary Care Services: A Pilot Cluster Randomized Clinical Trial. *JAMA Netw Open, 4*(11), e2131475. https://doi.org/10.1001/jamanetworkopen.2021.31475

Koseoglu, Z. (2022). Launch of the revised version on the Istanbul Protocol. *Torture, 32*(3), 89. https://doi.org/10.7146/torture.v32i3.133934

Kratzer, L., Knefel, M., Haselgruber, A., Heinz, P., Schennach, R., & Karatzias, T. (2022, Aug). Co-occurrence of severe PTSD, somatic symptoms and dissociation in a large sample of childhood trauma inpatients: a network analysis. *Eur Arch Psychiatry Clin Neurosci, 272*(5), 897-908. https://doi.org/10.1007/s00406-021-01342-z

Kubler-Ross, E. (1975, Jun). On death and dying. *Bull Am Coll Surg, 60*(6), 12, 15-17. https://www.ncbi.nlm.nih.gov/pubmed/10323918

Kuwert, P., Knaevelsrud, C., Rosenthal, J., Dudeck, M., Freyberger, H. J., & Spitzer, C. (2008, Nov). [Quality of life and sense of coherence in former German child soldiers of World War II]. *Psychiatr Prax, 35*(8), 399-403. https://doi.org/10.1055/s-2008-1067499 (Lebensqualitat und Koharenzgefuhl bei ehemaligen deutschen Kindersoldaten des Zweiten Weltkrieges.)

Kuwert, P., Spitzer, C., Rosenthal, J., & Freyberger, H. J. (2008, Oct). Trauma and post-traumatic stress symptoms in former German child soldiers of World War II. *Int Psychogeriatr, 20*(5), 1014-1018. https://doi.org/10.1017/S1041610208007035

Lam, P. C., Lewis-Fernandez, R., & Aggarwal, N. K. (2023, Feb 1). The Cultural Formulation Interview: Building the Case for Cultural Competence in Clinical Care. *Psychiatr Serv, 74*(2), 216-217.

https://doi.org/10.1176/appi.ps.202100650

Larsson, C., Axell, A. G., & Ersson, A. (2007, Aug). Confusion assessment method for the intensive care unit (CAM-ICU): translation, retranslation and validation into Swedish intensive care settings. *Acta Anaesthesiol Scand, 51*(7), 888-892. https://doi.org/10.1111/j.1399-6576.2007.01340.x

Lasater, M. E., Flemming, J., Bourey, C., Nemiro, A., & Meyer, S. R. (2022, Apr 21). School-based MHPSS interventions in humanitarian contexts: a realist review. *BMJ Open, 12*(4), e054856. https://doi.org/10.1136/bmjopen-2021-054856

Lemkin, R., & Bazyler, M. J. (2008). *Raphael Lemkin's dossier on the Armenian genocide : Turkish massacres of Armenians (manuscript from Raphael Lemkin's collection, American Jewish Historical Society)*. Center for Armenian Remembrance.

Lenferink, L. I. M., van den Munckhof, M. J. A., de Keijser, J., & Boelen, P. A. (2021). DSM-5-TR prolonged grief disorder and DSM-5 posttraumatic stress disorder are related, yet distinct: confirmatory factor analyses in traumatically bereaved people. *Eur J Psychotraumatol, 12*(1), 1-14. https://doi.org/10.1080/20008198.2021.2000131

Leung, J. G. (2023, Dec). Ethnopsychopharmacology: Clinical and scientific writing pearls. *Ment Health Clin, 13*(6), 276-288. https://doi.org/10.9740/mhc.2023.12.276

Lopes Cardozo, B., Kaiser, R., Gotway, C. A., & Agani, F. (2003, Aug). Mental health, social functioning, and feelings of hatred and revenge of Kosovar Albanians one year after the war in Kosovo. *J Trauma Stress, 16*(4), 351-360. https://doi.org/10.1023/A:1024413918346

Matiashova, L., Tsagkaris, C., Essar, M. Y., Romash, I. B., & Vus, V. I. (2022, Nov). Achilles in Ukraine: Concerns and priorities over the long-term implications of trauma. *Int J Health Plann Manage, 37*(6), 3369-3371. https://doi.org/10.1002/hpm.3562

McCann, J. P., Tipsword, J. M., Brake, C. A., & Badour, C. L. (2023, Oct). Trauma-Related Shame and Guilt as Prospective Predictors of Daily Mental Contamination and PTSD Symptoms in Survivors of Sexual Trauma. *J Interpers Violence, 38*(19-20), 11117-11137. https://doi.org/10.1177/08862605231179721

Meng, Y., Zhang, Y., Wang, S., Wu, S., Zhou, H., Ke, C., Qi, X., & Rainey, J. J. (2020, Jan). Lessons Learned in the Development of a Web-based Surveillance Reporting System and Dashboard to Monitor Acute Febrile Illnesses in Guangdong and Yunnan Provinces, China, 2017-2019. *Health Secur, 18*(S1), S14-S22. https://doi.org/10.1089/hs.2019.0079

Mental health: WHO minds the GAP. (2010, Oct 16). *Lancet, 376*(9749), 1274. https://doi.org/10.1016/S0140-6736(10)61898-3

Metz, C. J., & Metz, M. J. (2022, Mar 1). The benefits of incorporating active learning into online, asynchronous coursework in dental physiology. *Adv Physiol Educ, 46*(1), 11-20. https://doi.org/10.1152/advan.00110.2021

Meulenbroeks, R. (2020, Dec). Suddenly fully online: A case study of a blended university course moving online during the Covid-19 pandemic. *Heliyon, 6*(12), e05728. https://doi.org/10.1016/j.heliyon.2020.e05728

Mezzich, J. E., Kirmayer, L. J., Kleinman, A., Fabrega, H., Jr., Parron, D. L., Good, B. J., Lin, K. M., & Manson, S. M. (1999, Aug). The place of culture in DSM-IV. *J Nerv Ment Dis, 187*(8), 457-464. https://doi.org/10.1097/00005053-199908000-00001

Midgley, N., Guerrero-Tates, B., Mortimer, R., Edbrooke-Childs, J., Mechler, J., Lindqvist, K., Hajkowski, S., Leibovich, L., Martin, P., Andersson, G., Vlaescu, G., Lilliengren, P., Kitson, A., Butler-Wheelhouse, P., & Philips, B. (2021, Dec 9). The Depression: Online Therapy Study (D:OTS)-A Pilot Study of an Internet-Based Psychodynamic Treatment for Adolescents with Low Mood in the UK, in the Context of the COVID-19 Pandemic. *Int J Environ Res Public Health, 18*(24). https://doi.org/10.3390/ijerph182412993

Miller, M. (2002). Depression after cardiac transplant treated with interpersonal psychotherapy and paroxetine. *Am J Psychother, 56*(4), 555-561. https://doi.org/10.1176/appi.psychotherapy.2002.56.4.555

Mirzaei, S., Hardi, L., & Wenzel, T. (2011). How to combat torture if perpetrators are supported by a religious "justification". *Torture, 21*(3), 173-177. https://www.ncbi.nlm.nih.gov/pubmed/22057104

Mollica, R. F., Chernoff, M. C., Megan Berthold, S., Lavelle, J., Lyoo, I. K., & Renshaw, P. (2014, Oct). The mental health sequelae of traumatic head injury in South Vietnamese ex-political detainees who survived torture. *Compr Psychiatry, 55*(7), 1626-1638. https://doi.org/10.1016/j.comppsych.2014.04.014

Molloy, L., Beckett, P., Chidarikire, S., Merrick, T. T., Guha, M., & Patton, D. (2020, Nov 1). Culture, the Stigma of Mental Illness, and Young People. *J Psychosoc Nurs Ment Health Serv, 58*(11), 15-18. https://doi.org/10.3928/02793695-20201013-03

Moreno, A., & Grodin, M. A. (2002, May). Torture and its neurological sequelae. *Spinal Cord, 40*(5), 213-223. https://doi.org/10.1038/sj.sc.3101284

Muschalla, B., Rau, H., Willmund, G. D., & Knaevelsrud, C. (2018, Jan). Work disability in soldiers with posttraumatic stress disorder, post-traumatic embitterment disorder, and not-event-related common mental disorders. *Psychol Trauma, 10*(1), 30-35. https://doi.org/10.1037/tra0000293

Neumann, J. C., Berger, T., & Kizilhan, J. I. (2021, Nov 24). Development of a Questionnaire to Measure the Perceived Injustice of People Who Have Experienced Violence in War and Conflict Areas: Perceived Injustice Questionnaire (PIQ). *Int J Environ Res Public Health, 18*(23). https://doi.org/10.3390/ijerph182312357

Niederland, W. G. (1981). The survivor syndrome: further observations and dimensions. *J Am Psychoanal Assoc, 29*(2), 413-425. https://doi.org/10.1177/000306518102900207

Nolan, A. L., Petersen, C., Iacono, D., Mac Donald, C. L., Mukherjee, P., van der Kouwe, A., Jain, S., Stevens, A., Diamond, B. R., Wang, R., Markowitz, A. J., Fischl, B., Perl, D. P., Manley, G. T., Keene, C. D., Diaz-Arrastia, R., Edlow, B. L., & Investigators, T.-T. (2021, Jun 15). Tractography-Pathology Correlations in Traumatic Brain Injury: A TRACK-TBI Study. *J Neurotrauma, 38*(12), 1620-1631. https://doi.org/10.1089/neu.2020.7373

Novins, D. K., Bechtold, D. W., Sack, W. H., Thompson, J., Carter, D. R., & Manson, S. M. (1997, Sep). The DSM-IV Outline for Cultural Formulation: a critical demonstration with American Indian children. *J Am Acad Child Adolesc Psychiatry, 36*(9), 1244-1251. https://doi.org/10.1097/00004583-199709000-00017

O'Callaghan, P. (2014). Case study: ten lessons learned while carrying out a MHPSS intervention with war-affected children in the Democratic Republic of Congo in 2011. *Int J Emerg Ment Health, 16*(1), 241-245. https://doi.org/10.4172/1522-4821.1000103

Panagioti, M., Gooding, P. A., Taylor, P. J., & Tarrier, N. (2014, Jan). Perceived social support buffers the impact of PTSD symptoms on suicidal behavior: implications into suicide resilience research. *Compr Psychiatry, 55*(1), 104-112. https://doi.org/10.1016/j.comppsych.2013.06.004

Parandeh Afshar, P., Keshavarz, F., Salehi, M., Fakhri Moghadam, R., Khajoui, E., Nazari, F., & Dehghan, M. (2022, Jan). Health Literacy and Media Literacy: Is There Any Relation? *Community Health Equity Res Policy, 42*(2), 195-201. https://doi.org/10.1177/0272684X20972642

Peckl, P. (2007, Dec 19). ["The patient before was always healthy" -- the "war trembler" in the mirror of military hospital patient records of

German soldiers during First World War]. *Praxis (Bern 1994), 96*(51-52), 2075-2079. https://doi.org/10.1024/1661-8157.96.51.2075 ("Patient will fruher immer gesund gewesen sein"--der "Kriegszitterer" im Spiegel der Lazarettkrankenakten deutscher Soldaten im Ersten Weltkrieg.)

Penk, W. E., & Robinowitz, R. (1989, Sep). Post-traumatic stress disorder (PTSD): issues of utility, traumatogenicity, co-morbidity, teratogenicity vs. psychogenicity, ethnicity, "gendericity" and chronicity. An introduction. *J Clin Psychol, 45*(5), 688-690. https://doi.org/10.1002/1097-4679(198909)45:5<688::aid-jclp2270450502>3.0.co;2-w

Pentaris, P. (2012, 01/01). Death in the Modern Greek Culture. *Hawaii Pacific Journal of Social Work Practice, 5*, 126-131.

Perin, S., Lai, R., Diehl-Schmid, J., You, E., Kurz, A., Tensil, M., Wenz, M., Foertsch, B., & Lautenschlager, N. T. (2023, Jan-Dec). Online counselling for family carers of people with young onset dementia: The RHAPSODY-Plus pilot study. *Digit Health, 9*, 20552076231161962. https://doi.org/10.1177/20552076231161962

Peterson, C., Park, N., Pole, N., D'Andrea, W., & Seligman, M. E. (2008, Apr). Strengths of character and posttraumatic growth. *J Trauma Stress, 21*(2), 214-217. https://doi.org/10.1002/jts.20332

Phelan, S. M., Griffin, J. M., Hellerstedt, W. L., Sayer, N. A., Jensen, A. C., Burgess, D. J., & van Ryn, M. (2011, Jul). Perceived stigma, strain, and mental health among caregivers of veterans with traumatic brain injury. *Disabil Health J, 4*(3), 177-184. https://doi.org/10.1016/j.dhjo.2011.03.003

Quinn, N., Shulman, A., Knifton, L., & Byrne, P. (2011, Jan). The impact of a national mental health arts and film festival on stigma and recovery. *Acta Psychiatr Scand, 123*(1), 71-81. https://doi.org/10.1111/j.1600-0447.2010.01573.x

Quintana, D. A., Parker, J. R., Jordan, F. B., Tuggle, D. W., Mantor, P. C., & Tunell, W. P. (1997, Feb). The spectrum of pediatric injuries after a bomb blast. *J Pediatr Surg, 32*(2), 307-310; discussion 310-301. https://doi.org/10.1016/s0022-3468(97)90199-8

Raboni, M. R., Tufik, S., & Suchecki, D. (2006, Jul). Treatment of PTSD by eye movement desensitization reprocessing (EMDR) improves sleep quality, quality of life, and perception of stress. *Ann N Y Acad Sci, 1071*, 508-513. https://doi.org/10.1196/annals.1364.054

Raguram, R., & Weiss, M. (2004, Aug). Stigma and somatisation. *Br J Psychiatry, 185*, 174; author reply 174-175. https://doi.org/10.1192/bjp.185.2.174

Raguram, R., Weiss, M. G., Channabasavanna, S. M., & Devins, G. M. (1996, Aug). Stigma, depression, and somatization in South India. *Am J Psychiatry, 153*(8), 1043-1049. https://doi.org/10.1176/ajp.153.8.1043

Ray, S. L., & Vanstone, M. (2009, Jun). The impact of PTSD on veterans' family relationships: an interpretative phenomenological inquiry. *Int J Nurs Stud, 46*(6), 838-847. https://doi.org/10.1016/j.ijnurstu.2009.01.002

Resick, P. A., Straud, C. L., Wachen, J. S., LoSavio, S. T., Peterson, A. L., McGeary, D. D., Young-McCaughan, S., Taylor, D. J., Mintz, J., Consortium, S. S., & the Consortium to Alleviate, P. (2023). A comparison of the CAPS-5 and PCL-5 to assess PTSD in military and veteran treatment-seeking samples. *Eur J Psychotraumatol, 14*(2), 2222608. https://doi.org/10.1080/20008066.2023.2222608

Riaz, M. M. A., Nayyer, B., Lal, A., Nawaz, F. A., & Zil, E. A. A. (2023, Aug). Climate change and mental health: a call to action to include mental health and psychosocial support services (MHPSS) in the Pakistan flood crisis. *BJPsych Int, 20*(3), 56-58. https://doi.org/10.1192/bji.2023.13

Rosenfeld, J. V., & Ford, N. L. (2010, May). Bomb blast, mild traumatic brain injury and psychiatric morbidity: a review. *Injury, 41*(5), 437-443. https://doi.org/10.1016/j.injury.2009.11.018

Ruiz-White, I., Kramer, L., Philips, L., Wong, B., Lonergan, K., & Moreno, F. (2023, Jun 12). Racial and Ethnic Disparities in Physical and Mental Health Care and Clinical Trials. *J Clin Psychiatry, 84*(4). https://doi.org/10.4088/JCP.23ah14887

Sabin, L. L., Thulasingam, M., Carwile, M., Babu, S. P., Knudsen, S., Dong, L., Stephens, J., Fernandes, P., Cintron, C., Horsburgh, C. R., Salgame, P., Ellner, J. J., Sarkar, S., & Hochberg, N. S. (2022, Nov). 'People listen more to what actors say': A qualitative study of tuberculosis-related knowledge, behaviours, stigma, and potential interventions in Puducherry, India. *Glob Public Health, 17*(11), 2898-2910. https://doi.org/10.1080/17441692.2021.1990372

Sanchez-Carrion, R., Fernandez-Espejo, D., Junque, C., Falcon, C., Bargallo, N., Roig, T., Bernabeu, M., Tormos, J. M., & Vendrell, P. (2008, Nov 15). A longitudinal fMRI study of working memory in severe TBI patients with diffuse axonal injury. *Neuroimage, 43*(3), 421-429. https://doi.org/10.1016/j.neuroimage.2008.08.003

Sarapas, C., Cai, G., Bierer, L. M., Golier, J. A., Galea, S., Ising, M., Rein, T., Schmeidler, J., Muller-Myhsok, B., Uhr, M., Holsboer, F., Buxbaum, J. D., & Yehuda, R. (2011). Genetic markers for PTSD risk and resilience among survivors of the World Trade Center attacks. *Dis Markers, 30*(2-3), 101-110. https://doi.org/10.3233/DMA-2011-0764

Saymah, D., Tait, L., & Michail, M. (2015). An overview of the mental health system in Gaza: an assessment using the World Health Organization's Assessment Instrument for Mental Health Systems (WHO-AIMS). *Int J Ment Health Syst, 9*, 4. https://doi.org/10.1186/1752-4458-9-4

Schafer, S. K., Becker, N., King, L., Horsch, A., & Michael, T. (2019). The relationship between sense of coherence and post-traumatic stress: a meta-analysis. *Eur J Psychotraumatol, 10*(1), 1562839. https://doi.org/10.1080/20008198.2018.1562839

Seidler, G. H., & Wagner, F. E. (2006, Nov). Comparing the efficacy of EMDR and trauma-focused cognitive-behavioral therapy in the treatment of PTSD: a meta-analytic study. *Psychol Med, 36*(11), 1515-1522. https://doi.org/10.1017/S0033291706007963

Shakespeare-Finch, J., & Enders, T. (2008, Aug). Corroborating evidence of posttraumatic growth. *J Trauma Stress, 21*(4), 421-424. https://doi.org/10.1002/jts.20347

Shandera-Ochsner, A. L., Berry, D. T., Harp, J. P., Edmundson, M., Graue, L. O., Roach, A., & High, W. M., Jr. (2013). Neuropsychological effects of self-reported deployment-related mild TBI and current PTSD in OIF/OEF veterans. *Clin Neuropsychol, 27*(6), 881-907. https://doi.org/10.1080/13854046.2013.802017

Shay, J. (1994). *Achilles in Vietnam : combat trauma and the undoing of character*. Atheneum ;

Maxwell Macmillan Canada ; Maxwell Macmillan International.

Shin, J. H., & Yim, S. V. (2023, Aug). A Foundation for a "Cheerful Society": The Korean War and the Rise of Psychiatry. *Uisahak, 32*(2), 553-591. https://doi.org/10.13081/kjmh.2023.32.553

Shively, S. B., & Perl, D. P. (2012, May-Jun). Traumatic brain injury, shell shock, and posttraumatic stress disorder in the military--past, present, and future. *J Head Trauma Rehabil, 27*(3), 234-239. https://doi.org/10.1097/HTR.0b013e318250e9dd

Singh, S. K., Kumar, A., & Katyal, S. (2014, May-Aug). A terrorist bomb blast, a real challenge for any tertiary care health provider. *Anesth Essays Res, 8*(2), 229-232. https://doi.org/10.4103/0259-1162.134517

Sippel, L. M., Han, S., Watkins, L. E., Harpaz-Rotem, I., Southwick, S. M., Krystal, J. H., Olff, M., Sherva, R., Farrer, L. A., Kranzler, H. R., Gelernter, J., & Pietrzak, R. H. (2017, Nov). Oxytocin receptor gene polymorphisms, attachment, and PTSD: Results from the National

Health and Resilience in Veterans Study. *J Psychiatr Res, 94*, 139-147. https://doi.org/10.1016/j.jpsychires.2017.07.008

Skammeritz, S., Lindberg, L. G., Mortensen, E. L., Norredam, M., & Carlsson, J. (2020, Aug). Using the Cultural Formulation Interview in Denmark: Acceptability and clinical utility for medical doctors and migrant patients. *Transcult Psychiatry, 57*(4), 556-566. https://doi.org/10.1177/1363461520935673

Soldatos, C. R., Paparrigopoulos, T. J., Pappa, D. A., & Christodoulou, G. N. (2006, Aug 30). Early post-traumatic stress disorder in relation to acute stress reaction: an ICD-10 study among help seekers following an earthquake. *Psychiatry Res, 143*(2-3), 245-253. https://doi.org/10.1016/j.psychres.2005.05.018

Somasundaram, D. (2002, May 25). Child soldiers: understanding the context. *BMJ, 324*(7348), 1268-1271. https://doi.org/10.1136/bmj.324.7348.1268

Somasundaram, D. (2007, Oct 4). Collective trauma in northern Sri Lanka: a qualitative psychosocial-ecological study. *Int J Ment Health Syst, 1*(1), 5. https://doi.org/10.1186/1752-4458-1-5

Somasundaram, D. (2010, Jul 28). Collective trauma in the Vanni- a qualitative inquiry into the mental health of the internally displaced due to the civil war in Sri Lanka. *Int J Ment Health Syst, 4*, 22. https://doi.org/10.1186/1752-4458-4-22

Sorensen, H., Hansen, O. E., & Worm-Petersen, J. (1983, Nov 21). [Sailors during the war: 40 years later. Psychological and social sequelae - a pilot study]. *Ugeskr Laeger, 145*(47), 3685-3688. https://www.ncbi.nlm.nih.gov/pubmed/6659145 (Krigssejlere 40 ar efter. Psykiske og sociale folger - en pilotundersogelse.)

Southwell, B. G., Niederdeppe, J., Cappella, J. N., Gaysynsky, A., Kelley, D. E., Oh, A., Peterson, E. B., & Chou, W. S. (2019, Aug). Misinformation as a Misunderstood Challenge to Public Health. *Am J Prev Med, 57*(2), 282-285. https://doi.org/10.1016/j.amepre.2019.03.009

Stein, D. J. (1998, Dec). Psychiatric aspects of the Truth and Reconciliation Commission in South Africa. *Br J Psychiatry, 173*, 455-457. https://doi.org/10.1192/bjp.173.6.455

Stein, D. J., Schmidt, A., Bouwer, C., & Allan, A. (1997, Jun). The Truth and Reconciliation Commission and post-traumatic stress disorder. *S Afr Med J, 87*(6), 763. https://www.ncbi.nlm.nih.gov/pubmed/9254751

Stewart, A. E. (1999, Jun). Complicated bereavement and posttraumatic stress disorder following fatal car crashes: recommendations for death notification practice. *Death Stud, 23*(4), 289-321. https://doi.org/10.1080/074811899200984

Stompe, T., Ortwein-Swoboda, G., Chaudhry, H. R., Friedmann, A., Wenzel, T., & Schanda, H. (2001, Nov-Dec). Guilt and depression: a cross-cultural comparative study. *Psychopathology, 34*(6), 289-298. https://doi.org/10.1159/000049327

Summerfield, D. (1991, Nov 16). The rise of post-traumatic stress disorders. *BMJ, 303*(6812), 1271. https://doi.org/10.1136/bmj.303.6812.1271

Summerfield, D. (1998, Sep 12). Trauma, post-traumatic stress disorder, and war. *Lancet, 352*(9131), 911. https://doi.org/10.1016/S0140-6736(05)60057-8

Summerfield, D. (2002, Apr 13). ICD and DSM are contemporary cultural documents. *BMJ, 324*(7342), 914. https://doi.org/10.1136/bmj.324.7342.914/b

Summit, R. C. (1989, Jun). The centrality of victimization. Regaining the focal point of recovery for survivors of child sexual abuse. *Psychiatr Clin North Am, 12*(2), 413-430. https://www.ncbi.nlm.nih.gov/pubmed/2664733

Svingen, E. (2023, Jul). PTSD and crime propensity: Stress systems, brain structures, and the nature of the relationship. *Heliyon, 9*(7), e18381. https://doi.org/10.1016/j.heliyon.2023.e18381

Swartz, L., & Drennan, G. (2000, Aug-Nov). The cultural construction of healing in the Truth and Reconciliation Commission: implications for mental health practice. *Ethn Health, 5*(3-4), 205-213. https://doi.org/10.1080/713667455

Sznaider, N. (2011). *Jewish memory and the cosmopolitan order : Hannah Arendt and the Jewish condition*. Polity. https://doi.org/99943620923

Tanev, K. S., Pentel, K. Z., Kredlow, M. A., & Charney, M. E. (2014). PTSD and TBI co-morbidity: scope, clinical presentation and treatment options. *Brain Inj, 28*(3), 261-270. https://doi.org/10.3109/02699052.2013.873821

Tanne, J. H. (2010, Mar 9). US pro-life groups ask black women to avoid abortion, calling it genocide. *BMJ, 340*, c1366. https://doi.org/10.1136/bmj.c1366

Tatz, C. (2001). Confronting Australian genocide. *Aborig Hist, 25*, 16-36. https://www.ncbi.nlm.nih.gov/pubmed/19514155

Te Brake, H., Willems, A., Steen, C., & Duckers, M. (2022, Mar 6). Appraising Evidence-Based Mental Health and Psychosocial Support (MHPSS) Guidelines-PART I: A Systematic Review on Methodological Quality Using AGREE-HS. *Int J Environ Res Public Health, 19*(5). https://doi.org/10.3390/ijerph19053107

Tischler, L., Brand, S. R., Stavitsky, K., Labinsky, E., Newmark, R., Grossman, R., Buchsbaum, M. S., & Yehuda, R. (2006, Jul). The relationship between hippocampal volume and declarative memory in a population of combat veterans with and without PTSD. *Ann N Y Acad Sci, 1071*, 405-409. https://doi.org/10.1196/annals.1364.031

Troiani, J. E. (2012, Mar-Apr). Fighting for hearts and minds. *Behav Healthc, 32*(2), 10-13. https://www.ncbi.nlm.nih.gov/pubmed/22550784

Turner, L. (2003, Sep). Zones of consensus and zones of conflict: questioning the "common morality" presumption in bioethics. *Kennedy Inst Ethics J, 13*(3), 193-218. https://doi.org/10.1353/ken.2003.0023

Turner, R. J., & Avison, W. R. (2003, Dec). Status variations in stress exposure: implications for the interpretation of research on race, socioeconomic status, and gender. *J Health Soc Behav, 44*(4), 488-505. https://www.ncbi.nlm.nih.gov/pubmed/15038145

van Denderen, M., de Keijser, J., Gerlsma, C., Huisman, M., & Boelen, P. A. (2014, Nov-Dec). Revenge and psychological adjustment after homicidal loss. *Aggress Behav, 40*(6), 504-511. https://doi.org/10.1002/ab.21543

Ventriglio, A., Ayonrinde, O., & Bhugra, D. (2016, Jan). Relevance of culture-bound syndromes in the 21st century. *Psychiatry Clin Neurosci, 70*(1), 3-6. https://doi.org/10.1111/pcn.12359

Vindevogel, S., Broekaert, E., & Derluyn, I. (2013, Aug). "It helps me transform in my life from the past to the new": the meaning of resources for former child soldiers. *J Interpers Violence, 28*(12), 2413-2436. https://doi.org/10.1177/0886260513479031

Volkan, V., & Javakhishvili, J. D. (2022, Jun). Invasion of Ukraine: Observations on Leader-Followers Relationships. *Am J Psychoanal, 82*(2), 189-209. https://doi.org/10.1057/s11231-022-09349-8

Volkan, V. D. (1980, Apr). Narcissistic personality organization and "reparative" leadership. *Int J Group Psychother, 30*(2), 131-152. https://doi.org/10.1080/00207284.1980.11491677

Volkan, V. D. (1987). Psychological concepts useful in the building of political foundations between nations: Track II diplomacy. *J Am Psychoanal Assoc, 35*(4), 903-935. https://doi.org/10.1177/000306518703500406

Volkan, V. D. (2019, Jun). Large-Group Identity, Who Are We Now? Leader-Follower Relationships and Societal-Political Divisions. *Am J Psychoanal, 79*(2), 139-155. https://doi.org/10.1057/s11231-019-09186-2

Volkan, V. D. (2021, Jun). Trauma, Prejudice, Large-Group Identity and Psychoanalysis. *Am J Psychoanal, 81*(2), 137-154.

https://doi.org/10.1057/s11231-021-09285-z

Wagner, B., Brand, J., Schulz, W., & Knaevelsrud, C. (2012, Jul). Online working alliance predicts treatment outcome for posttraumatic stress symptoms in Arab war-traumatized patients. *Depress Anxiety, 29*(7), 646-651. https://doi.org/10.1002/da.21962

Wenzel, T., Frewer, A., & Mirzaei, S. (2015). The DSM 5 and the Istanbul Protocol: Diagnosis of psychological sequels of torture. *Torture, 25*(1), 51-61. https://www.ncbi.nlm.nih.gov/pubmed/26021347

Wenzel, T., Griengl, H., Stompe, T., Mirzaei, S., & Kieffer, W. (2000, Nov-Dec). Psychological disorders in survivors of torture: exhaustion, impairment and depression. *Psychopathology, 33*(6), 292-296. https://doi.org/10.1159/000029160

Wenzel, T., Kizilhan, J. I., Alksiri, R., Dorfler, D., Messerschmidt, E. J., & Chen, A. F. (2021, Aug 24). FGM and Restorative Justice-A Challenge for Developing Countries and for Refugee Women. *Int J Environ Res Public Health, 18*(17). https://doi.org/10.3390/ijerph18178913

Werner, E. E. (2012, May). Children and war: risk, resilience, and recovery. *Dev Psychopathol, 24*(2), 553-558. https://doi.org/10.1017/S0954579412000156

Wilson, J. P. (1994, Oct). The historical evolution of PTSD diagnostic criteria: from Freud to DSM-IV. *J Trauma Stress, 7*(4), 681-698. https://doi.org/10.1007/BF02103015

Wilson, S. R., Rodda, S., Lubman, D. I., Manning, V., & Yap, M. B. H. (2017, Jul). How online counselling can support partners of individuals with problem alcohol or other drug use. *J Subst Abuse Treat, 78*, 56-62. https://doi.org/10.1016/j.jsat.2017.04.009

Wisco, B. E., Marx, B. P., Holowka, D. W., Vasterling, J. J., Han, S. C., Chen, M. S., Gradus, J. L., Nock, M. K., Rosen, R. C., & Keane, T. M. (2014, Apr). Traumatic brain injury, PTSD, and current suicidal ideation among Iraq and Afghanistan U.S. veterans. *J Trauma Stress, 27*(2), 244-248. https://doi.org/10.1002/jts.21900

Woodward, S. H., Kaloupek, D. G., Streeter, C. C., Kimble, M. O., Reiss, A. L., Eliez, S., Wald, L. L., Renshaw, P. F., Frederick, B. B., Lane, B., Sheikh, J. I., Stegman, W. K., Kutter, C. J., Stewart, L. P., Prestel, R. S., & Arsenault, N. J. (2006, Apr). Hippocampal volume, PTSD, and alcoholism in combat veterans. *Am J Psychiatry, 163*(4), 674-681. https://doi.org/10.1176/ajp.2006.163.4.674

Yates, R., Anderson, P. J., Lee, K. J., Doyle, L. W., Cheong, J. L. Y., Pace, C. C., Spittle, A. J., Spencer-Smith, M., & Treyvaud, K. (2022, Mar 5). Maternal Mental Health Disorders Following Very Preterm

Birth at 5 Years Post-Birth. *J Pediatr Psychol, 47*(3), 327-336. https://doi.org/10.1093/jpepsy/jsab101

Yeh, P. H., Wang, B., Oakes, T. R., French, L. M., Pan, H., Graner, J., Liu, W., & Riedy, G. (2014, Jun). Postconcussional disorder and PTSD symptoms of military-related traumatic brain injury associated with compromised neurocircuitry. *Hum Brain Mapp, 35*(6), 2652-2673. https://doi.org/10.1002/hbm.22358

Yue, J. K., Burke, J. F., Upadhyayula, P. S., Winkler, E. A., Deng, H., Robinson, C. K., Pirracchio, R., Suen, C. G., Sharma, S., Ferguson, A. R., Ngwenya, L. B., Stein, M. B., Manley, G. T., & Tarapore, P. E. (2017, Jul 25). Selective Serotonin Reuptake Inhibitors for Treating Neurocognitive and Neuropsychiatric Disorders Following Traumatic Brain Injury: An Evaluation of Current Evidence. *Brain Sci, 7*(8). https://doi.org/10.3390/brainsci7080093

Zawadzki, B., Popiel, A., Cyniak-Cieciura, M., Jakubowska, B., & Praglowska, E. (2015, Jan-Feb). [Diagnosis of Posttraumatic Stress Disorder (PTSD) by the Structured Clinical Interview SCID-I]. *Psychiatr Pol, 49*(1), 159-169. https://doi.org/10.12740/PP/32214 (Diagnoza pourazowego zaburzenia stresowego (PTSD) za pomoca ustrukturalizowanego wywiadu klinicznego SCID-I.)

Zheng, X., Chung, J. O., & Woo, B. K. (2016, Apr). Exploring the Impact of a Culturally Tailored Short Film in Modifying Dementia Stigma Among Chinese Americans: A Pilot Study. *Acad Psychiatry, 40*(2), 372-374. https://doi.org/10.1007/s40596-015-0397-7

Zuair, A. A., & Sopory, P. (2022, Jan). Effects of Media Health Literacy School-Based Interventions on Adolescents' Body Image Concerns, Eating Concerns, and Thin-Internalization Attitudes: A Systematic Review and Meta-Analysis. *Health Commun, 37*(1), 20-28. https://doi.org/10.1080/10410236.2020.1813954

CHAPTER 2

PSYCHOTHERAPY TRAINING AND PROFESSIONALIZATION: A DEVELOPING FIELD

THOMAS WENZEL AND JAN KIZILHAN

In this book chapter we want to follow up further on the history and practice of possible interventions to the problems and some aspects of their possible use in countries like Iraq, while the next chapters will analyze the social and health care situation in this country and focus on the Duhok project history, details and outcomes.

Historically, pioneers in psychotherapy implemented training which typically reflected the specific forms of psychotherapy that they developed. Sigmund Freud's informal method of teaching and providing "self" therapy (referred to as "Lehranalyse", treatment of the therapists own neurotic tendencies, also to learn from example) is a good example of this approach. While it might have been appropriate at the time, his informal approach is by now viewed rather critically and has been replaced by more formalized settings.

Psychotherapy as a profession has developed since these pioneering times, and comprehensive curricula with multiple controlled certification levels have been developed over recent decades. "Training the trainer" (ToT) models have been at the core of these developments, and while they have been validated in recent research (Wilfley et al., 2020), they require further inquiry. Various training models were recently reviewed in a meta-review by Frank et al. (2020), who explored the challenges of providing efficient training in evidence-based interventions (EBI). Frank proposes that training models should be classified into several categories: "workshop only (an "in-person" time-limited training opportunity that focuses on a single intervention topic), workshop plus consultation (workshop plus additional expert consultation/supervision after conclusion of the initial training), online training (training conducted via an online platform with either asynchronous [self-paced] or synchronous learning, with or without consultation), ToT (an expert trainer trains a set of local trainers who in turn will train local therapists, alternatively called a "cascade" model of training), and intensive training (defined as at least 20 hours of training plus two or more additional training components, such as consultation, direct observation of practice, or learning collaboratives)" (Frank et al., 2020). The authors reported that there has been a significant increase in research on the issue. They also drew attention to the complexities of this field and the important, but often unclear role of the trainer's social and cultural background and personal characteristics Frank et al., 2020)

Psychotherapists face numerous challenges in their work that will be summarized, but not detailed, in this book. These challenges include, but are not limited to, issues that arise when applying European or US-based models in regions with low healthcare resources. The use of EBIs in therapist training and clinical practice should adhere to strict guidelines, such as incorporating self-reflection, supervision and monitoring treatment practices. These strict standards are typically part of comprehensive education programs in university settings. Therefore, the project presented in this book opted for a university setting that integrated general basic education in psychology and mental health, to ensure a high standard of training.

Within the context of developing countries and crisis settings, several aspects pertaining to the development of psychotherapy training and its implementation should be discussed. These are listed below.

1) *Evidence base*. Psychotherapy research has in some respects been lagging behind other sciences and was only established as an objective discipline in recent decades. This is probably due to the difficulty in balancing different conceptual models, and individualized or "person-centered" factors, with the need for standardization in scientific research models. These scientific requirements have probably favored positivist approaches like Behavioral Therapy, against "humanistic" approaches like Positive Psychotherapy or psychoanalytic approaches (Kizilhan & Wenzel, 2020). Support for therapies like Cognitive Behavior Therapy (CBT) may be due to the fact that they require less complex resourcing and less time for training. Many projects and research studies in the international literature focus on post-conflict psychological problems and training programs aimed at treating mood disorders (Cunningham & Shapiro, 2018). These projects and studies usually focus on CBT and similar therapeutic models. Scoping reviews, such as the one by Frank et al. (2020) mentioned earlier, suggest that training in evidence-based therapies in practice often involves a very low number of training hours. There is in many international projects typically no clear definition of participant selection, supervised practice, or

self-therapy (self-reflection), which are part of common training programs in European countries. These standards are outlined, for instance, in the requirements of the European Certificate of Psychotherapy by the European Association for Psychotherapy (Frank et al., 2020) or similar standards.

2) *The considerable differences between cultures*, especially considering movements towards globalization in healthcare (Kizilhan, 2014, 2017), as also discussed in preceding chapters. Early pioneers, especially in psychoanalytic movements, are viewed with skepticism today because they often used their new treatment models without the benefit of rigorous transcultural research which is available in disciplines like anthropology today. Their approaches therefore often lacked critical scrutiny when applied to different cultures. A similar situation can be observed in our experiences in disaster and post-conflict regions, where newly developed treatment forms, which may not yet be evidence-based, are promoted uncritically across vastly different cultures. These new treatments, which are sometimes not even tested, and well established in their home countries, are transferred from one culture, are often US-based, and promoted in other regions, as noted, without sufficient scrutiny. The methodologies used in these studies are inappropriate in our experience, and would not be accepted in the US or Europe. Publications are sometimes used to promote, rather than evaluate, new short-lived projects in critical regions. It is a sad fact that most training curricula either completely neglect or sideline cultural and community aspects (Mathias et al., 2024), and those who want to train as psychotherapists from "third world" countries face various barriers (Madu et al., 1998), while they would urgently be needed by local health care services.

3) *Professional psychotherapy is trying to keep up with other developments in healthcare*, and many countries are moving towards mainstream processes of embedding both training and research also in psychotherapy into university structures, with clearly defined curricula and priorities. This process of embedding psychotherapy training and research into university structures was developed with the intention of countering the common exclusion of psychotherapy training from low-cost or free, more "democratic" public institutions. Traditionally, psychotherapy training has been offered by training organizations of different schools and was highly expensive for trainees. This should be viewed as a barrier and a potential risk of a lack of objective control over the quality of training outcomes. These problems are crucial to consider when introducing psychotherapy training into international collaborations and into mental health research in

developing countries, especially where resources are low in (post) conflict environments (Kienzler, 2019a, 2019b; Lin et al., 2023). Unfortunately, many "quick" interventions in crisis situations focus on the lowest standards of training models, which are not evidence-based, not comprehensively embedded, and focus only on selected issues, without consideration of sustainability and long-term service delivery.

Considering these three challenges, it is not surprising that in many countries, psychotherapy training and practice are not fully or officially recognized by healthcare insurance systems (Pasternack, 1977) and legislations. In the public view, their tasks are often taken up by medical doctors (Rennie, 1947). This book will not delve into the long-standing discussion of which professionals should be trained in and offer psychotherapy (Kirkpatrick et al., 1949; Lott, 1952; Luchines, 1949), especially when we keep in mind that medical doctors can rarely provide these time-intensive services in developing countries. The stigma of mental health problems, their treatment, and of service providers and the counter-productive competition with other health care professions is also firmly entrenched in many traditional societies, as discussed earlier in this book.

Projects like the Duhok/Iraq example presented in this book (Beckmann et al., 2022) - which was successfully implemented in a country with almost all of the challenges mentioned in these chapters - need to follow a comprehensive strategic plan, which considers potential challenges, and especially interdisciplinary and cultural factors. One of the most important interdisciplinary aspects of mental health services in post-conflict areas and regions affected by mass violence involves the relationship between law and society.

Therapeutic Justice in the context of individual and group mental health: International comparisons and Iraq

As mentioned in prior chapters, a key topic which emerged through our project was justice and accountability. For the feeling of justice to be achieved, it may initially involve an aspect of punishment and retribution. However, it is also based on a desire for security and the guarantee that "it should never happen again." These were issues which came up in the project preparation and treatment efforts (Kizilhan & Neumann, 2020; Neumann et al., 2021) and have also been explored independently by Matyas, Akhavan et al., with a focus on the Yazidi in the region (Matyas et al., 2020). Akhavan et al. drew attention to these problems and highlighted that trials in Iraq tend to proceed according to local anti-terror laws with "no legislation in place to incorporate international crimes into domestic law". This last concept reflects again revenge-based and punitive models (Matyas et al., 2020). The International Criminal Court (ICC's) approach of seeking justice may be even more difficult to implement with non-state actors such as ISIS, despite similar proceedings against Kony and the "LRA" terrorist group in Uganda[39]. In Northern Iraq processes for justice might not be sufficiently supported by the UN Security Council and the Iraqi national government. Therefore, the UN installed the UNITAD investigative team with Security Council Resolution 2379, on September 21st, 2017 (Gilmore, 2018). Unfortunately, their mandate was recently terminated. The UNITAD action included a psychological sub-team, which needed to elicit as much relevant information from victims about perpetrators and their violations. Collecting information from survivors was challenging for the team as this can create additional distress, suffering, and a worsening of trauma-related reactions in survivors. This challenge has also been reported in other human rights projects.

This important process was complemented by the capacity building of the professional trauma-focused psychotherapy in the Duhok project. This project also aimed to support the efforts of other projects in the extended Sinjar region, which had been exposed to the most extreme ISIS atrocities, including UNIDATs important work and similar activities. It should be noted that the issue of secondary victimization in the context of testimony-taking and therapeutic justice was also recently addressed by international guidelines, such as the World Psychiatric Association (WPA) Section (Wenzel T, 2023), the EU "Victims' Directive"[40], and an ICC[41] Protocol ("on the Vulnerability Assessment and Support Procedure used to facilitate the testimony of vulnerable witnesses"). Further, all victim groups should receive special consideration as vulnerable groups according to the EU reception guidelines for refugees and asylum seekers[42].

---

[39] See for example https://www.aljazeera.com/news/2022/11/24/icc-prosecutor-seeks-charges-against-fugitive-warlord-kony, accessed 2.2.2024

[40] Directive 2012/29/EU of the European Parliament and of the Council of 25 October 2012 establishing minimum standards on the rights, support and protection of victims of crime, https://eur-lex.europa.eu/legal-content/EN/ TXT/ ?uri=CELEX:32012L0029

[41] See https://www.icc-cpi.int/sites/default/files/RelatedRecords/CR2014_ 10208.PDF, accessed 9.2.2024

[42] DIRECTIVE 2013/33/EU OF THE EUROPEAN PARLIAMENT AND OF THE COUNCIL of 26 June 2013 laying down standards for the reception of applicants

Increased understanding of the risks to the psychological health of witnesses involved in legal investigations reiterates the need for training health care personnel to be available for survivors, especially in countries with limited health care structures. The UN Convention against Torture (CAT), for example, underlines the responsibility of all states to provide redress for victims of torture, which should include state-of-the-art psychotherapy for survivors[43]. The UN (CAT) specifically states in article 14, that: "1. Each State Party shall ensure in its legal system that the victim of an act of torture obtains redress and has an enforceable right to fair and adequate compensation, including the means for as full rehabilitation as possible. In the event of the death of the victim as a result of an act of torture, his dependents shall be entitled to compensation."

The above documents indirectly also highlight the long-neglected need for sustainable parallel strategies in law, social, and health systems in areas where massive human rights violations have occurred. To achieve this, interdisciplinary approaches are a necessity. Standards might be needed to guide such interdisciplinary strategies, including the work of health care professionals. Two standards may be of particular relevance in this context. The Minnesota protocol[44] guides the forensic examination of bodies of persons killed as part of suspected severe human rights violations. The recently updated Istanbul protocol[45] (Revised United Nations Manual on the Effective Prevention and Investigation of Extra-legal, Arbitrary and Summary Executions) was developed by an international interdisciplinary expert team and accepted by the UN General Assembly in its original version. This standard deals as also mentioned before with the examination of living and usually psychologically traumatized survivors (Akar et al., 2014; Iacopino et al., 2022; Koseoglu, 2022; Wenzel et al., 2015). It underlines the need for a good physical forensic examination but also the central role of a psychological assessment (p.115 ff of the protocol). The presence of these protocols underlines the need for capacity building in forensic and mental health fields, as discussed in the context of

---

for international protection (recast), see https://eur-lex.europa.eu/legal-content/EN/TXT/PDF/?uri=CELEX:32013L0033&from=EN, accessed 20.12.2023

[43] https://www.ohchr.org/en/instruments-mechanisms/instruments/convention-against-torture-and-other-cruel-inhuman-or-degrading accessed 20.12.2023

[44] The Revised United Nations Manual on the Effective Prevention and Investigation of Extra-legal, Arbitrary and Summary Executions, accessed 20.1.2024

[45] https://www.ohchr.org/en/publications/policy-and-methodological-publications/istanbul-protocol-manual-effective-0

UNITAD in Iraq. The project team kept in contact and collaborated with UNITAD.

Neumann and Kizilhan (2021) have developed, tested, and applied a "Perceived Injustice Questionnaire". The questionnaire that could provide important information on the perception of justice by victims and emotional factors related to this issue was consequently translated into other languages and tested with similar groups, such as the Uighurs in a project by Munich University (LMU).

Across society and communities, a transitional justice process may be required, as proposed earlier. It might require a profound interdisciplinary understanding of cultural, legal, and psychological factors. The often non-retributive approach applied in many traditional societies (Caparos et al., 2020) focuses on recovering harmony in communities and, if possible, reintegrating perpetrators. This has become an important model not only in examples such as in the Acholi culture of Uganda (Baines, 2010; Pham et al., 2010), but for the concept of "transitional" justice in general (Wenzel et al., 2021).

Universities, governmental and non-governmental organizations, but especially local communities and the public, should be included in the process of therapeutic justice, to ensure an adequate strategy that addresses actual needs and the respective cultural and historical environments. It is only under these conditions that acceptance and an effective outcome can be expected.

In many cultures, institutions or strategies exist to help people cope with crises, such as bereavement when a family or community member has died or has been killed and justice in this context. These traditional justice institutions have been used after mass violence but require a comprehensive understanding of cultural factors. This was highlighted by Mwaka et al. in the context of reconstruction, healing, and transitional justice (Baines, 2010) in Africa. It is also illustrated by the mixed results of using traditional rituals in the aftermath of mass violence within the transitional justice framework (Caparos et al., 2020). Regardless of the research results on different models, interventions are needed to restore trust and security after mass violence and human rights violations.

Many survivors, their families, and communities expect a general feeling of trust in a binding "contrat social" (Avruch, 2010; Kaplan, 2014), as outlined by Jaques Rousseau. They also expect predictability, fairness, and potentially provisions for retribution. However, even within populations, victims' needs and expectations around justice as a healing factor may widely differ. As part of a larger study with different minority survivors with different religious backgrounds, Matyas, Akhavan et al. (REF) conducted a study using unstructured, in-depth interviews with a group of 50 women who had been held in captivity by ISIL/DAESH terror groups. The author reported that 98.71% of the participants indicated that they desire to seek justice for the crimes committed by ISIL. The interviews also explored subjective needs and interpretation of models for such justice. The study yielded a list which demonstrates the diversity of possible expectations the women had for justice. The list included: "(i) revenge and compensation, (ii) fair trial of the perpetrators followed by punishment, if convicted, (iii) healing wounds by sharing their experiences at the hands of ISIL with the world, (iv) international protection against further harm, and (v) international recognition of the crimes committed against "us" (meaning the group to which the respondents belonged)". The results of this study further demonstrated that perceptions of justice can differ greatly between religious groups, such as Yazidi, Christians, and other denominations.

In Iraq, processes towards justice are difficult. This is partially due to the diversity of ethnic groups with their own religions, history, and traditions. The process is further complicated by unclear legislation which is still under development, and the need to coordinate and agree on this legislation between the multi-religious Kurdish region and the government in Baghdad. In the Sinjar region, for example, Sunni denomination neighbors, allegedly colluded with Sunni ISIS terrorist groups (non-state actors with multiple alliances) in the persecution and abduction of Yazidi women, also described separately in this book. This led to mistrust and fear in survivors as outlined above to return home to traditional villages; they preferred to stay in refugee camps, which are becoming more and more permanent. This could be attributed to the lack of transitional justice and failure to re-establish expectations of safety. Whether the UNITAD process can contribute to a long-term solution remains to be seen, as necessary as it might be.

So far, the subjective perception of injustice in psychotherapy has scarcely been dealt with. It is an important topic that needs to be investigated in more detail, as proposed also by Kizilhan and Neumann (2020). Examples in other post-conflict zones demonstrate that an advanced understanding and independent psychological impact evaluation would be important in this new field, which has been pioneered by the "Truth- and Reconciliation Committees" in post-apartheid South Africa, for example. Insights and findings from this setting have been taken up by several publications (Allan & Allan, 2000; American Academy of Pediatrics Board of, 2020; Graybill, 2001; McGibbon, 2019; Spenceley, 2016; Swartz & Drennan, 2000). While the impacts of the Committees were not without controversies, some authors have found additional benefits. For example, Graybill (2001) underlined the importance of justice for the development of women's human rights as well. Allan and Allan (2000) concluded their recent analysis by emphasizing the therapeutic potential of legislators emphasizing truth, reconciliation, stability, and restorative justice within the Truth and Reconciliation Commission (TRC) framework. They highlighted that while these legislative aspects enhanced the TRC's capacity to promote healing, certain features of the procedure and the Promotion of National Unity and Reconciliation Act (1995), limited its therapeutic effectiveness (Allan & Allan, 2000).

An additional challenge is the limited effectiveness of international courts and institutions in monitoring and enforcing human rights and humanitarian law standards, especially when perpetrators are non-state actors. This has been examined in the Iraq context by Saman, O. (1) and in a Master's thesis by Dinnayai, M. (2), as well as by other authors. This complex issue will be explored in-depth in a forthcoming publication by our group. In a recent publication, Kizilhan et al. explored the interaction between post-conflict development in a traditional culture and society with a strict caste system, with internationalized human rights concepts (3).

The project as seen from the general considerations mentioned in the earlier parts of this book

In this subchapter we will reflect on some aspects of the project following the earlier considerations, while the next chapter by the project leader, will take up the question of possible strategies in the project, that are also of relevance to planning and support in similar regions, "beyond MHPSS", followed by a more detailed history of the project implementation. We will further contribute an end-of project summary review and evaluation in one of the final chapters of this book.

Considerations for the project - implementing solutions for challenges

In preparation for the project, a comprehensive evaluation of available resources and challenges was conducted, which involved interviews, collaboration with key stakeholders on different levels, and also affected individuals in multiple camps. Relevant stakeholders included political stakeholders like the Kurdish Regional Autonomy Region representatives, religious community leaders, Universities, and health care providers. The results of the needs analysis are presented in a separate chapter on "Health care, social structure and history of Iraq in the context of war impact and reconstruction". A discussion on the MHPSS model (Marshall, 2022), which have been applied in similar disaster regions, were analyzed and relevant aspects were adapted by the project team (described by Kizilhan et al. in this book).

It was decided that professional University-based psychotherapy training, following developments in European countries like Germany and Austria, would be the best approach for providing a local team which was as sustainable as possible for the long-term improvement of public health in the area. Considering the specific challenges present in the country, added value was urgently needed above and beyond the numerous short-term services and projects in the region. The project model could also be tested, evaluated, and adapted to other regions, if successful.

As explained in more detail in the chapter offering a "Description of the pilot project", the Kurdish Regional Autonomy Region was chosen as the location for the planned project, due to several factors:

1) The relatively stable administration and positive development of the legal, social, and economic situation in the Kurdish Autonomous Region (as compared to other regions of Iraq).

2) The large mental GAP (WHO) in this neglected region (Mayor, 2008; Pinchuk et al., 2021) due to multiple interrelated factors, including stigma, political strategies, discrimination against minorities, and low resources, with extremely limited or non-existent access to professional, state-of-the-art trauma and mental health treatment for most population groups.

3) The strong contact between the University of Duhok, which led locally, and German universities.

4) The extensive violence experienced by the population, especially by minorities such as the Yazidi (Kizilhan et al., 2023; Kizilhan et al., 2020; Kizilhan & Noll-Hussong, 2017). This group had already been exposed to multiple events of extreme violence in earlier regimes, leading to greater vulnerability associated with transgenerational impact of genocides and persecution.

In the consultation, coordination, and preparation process, the project leaders identified and addressed several key issues, which were complex and challenging for a joint research effort with local stakeholders. To summarize, the situation was complicated by several factors, similar to situations in other countries of the region and the developing world. These factors included, but were not limited to:

- The lack of infrastructure and public transportation, which creates barriers to help-seeking;
- The stigma against acknowledging and seeking treatment for psychological trauma and mental health needs in general;
- Unproductive competition and lack of strategic integration of efforts between national and international NGOs in disaster regions (Nashwan et al., 2023; Sewordor et al., 2019);
- Creating understanding and coordination with local authorities.

Many projects in the field tend to focus on the delivery of services directly to survivors by experts from other countries, cultures, and foreign NGOs. Building sustainable, long-term, professional capacity is frequently neglected, either because the local population is not trusted, in worst cases because of post-colonialist bias, or because there is too much focus on maintaining the international NGOs. Further, the issue with many of these activities lies in the preferred use of insufficiently evidence-based and untested new therapy models. Are these models being applied uncritically from completely different cultures with different priorities? There is a need for a long-term sustainable model that prioritizes the needs of the local populations, especially as international support eventually fades out. Our careful preparatory steps identified the few existing resources available within the local context, but also highlighted needs that were not met. These unmet needs already existed before the crisis and attacks of ISIS/DAESH but were exacerbated by the multi-level, direct impact of traumatizing events such as abduction, sexual abuse, torture, and murder in the local population. These experiences were especially prominent for the Yazidi women.

As such, the project team decided to focus on ensuring long-term capacity building in the area, despite the insufficient resources. The team aimed to provide professional mental health experts, services, and specific culturally-sensitive trauma-focused psychotherapy. This approach followed international trends, especially in European countries with a high level of psychotherapy services and training. Specific factors were also considered for developing regions, as explored by Madu et al. (1998) in a careful analysis of the use of psychotherapy in African countries. The project concentrated on training and training trainers in this area, with the addition of internationally supervised clinical practice.

Cognitive behavioral therapy was selected as a key therapy for several reasons, including:

1) The solid evidence-base for CBT, which has been recently updated with a new focus on culture and trauma-focused modification of basic concepts (Johnson et al., 2024; Kananian et al., 2021; Naeem et al., 2021; Praptomojati et al., 2024);
2) Following the observations of the team, and after consultation with local experts, a culturally adapted CBT approach was seen as fitting for the local cultures;
3) Easy-to-adapt teaching models and strategies were available, including existing training materials and other resources which could easily be adapted for everyday mental health problems, as well as more complex treatment of trauma-related or other mental health GAP disorders.

The project could also benefit from the existing networks of trainers from the German partner universities, who joined the collaboration with the local partner university (The University of Duhok) from the beginning. From the outset, the team recognized that the local group of students should be "trained as trainers" to ensure an ongoing, sustainable future for the project, even after the their own education was complete. Feedback from the first pilot training phase would be used to further adapt, modify or improve the training model. Feedback would also be used to improve the transcultural competence of the international training team.

The project further considered the recommendations outlined in existing MHPSS guidelines, and related discussions (Marshall, 2022). These recommendations were adapted based on the results of preparatory consultations with all local stakeholders and the comprehensive country analyses conducted in the first planning phase.

The preparation phase also included the development of a teaching curriculum between all stakeholders, which was checked for compliance with international professional standards (German in this case). After the preparation phase, a selection process began to identify motivated and competent participants for the first year of training.

The training curriculum was, as noted before, based on the German model of professional psychotherapy training and adapted to existing local resources and standards in consultation with the local university, local healthcare stakeholders, local and international NGOs active in the region, and prospective students. The training curriculum is outlined separately in this book. It addresses most of the challenges listed in the first part of this book as part of a comprehensive strategy.

References

Akar, F. A., Arbel, R., Benninga, Z., Dia, M. A., & Steiner-Birmanns, B. (2014, Mar). The Istanbul protocol (manual on the effective investigation and documentation of torture and other cruel, inhuman or degrading treatment or punishment): implementation and education in Israel. *Isr Med Assoc J, 16*(3), 137-141. https://www.ncbi.nlm.nih.gov/pubmed/24761699

Allan, A., & Allan, M. M. (2000). The South African truth and reconciliation commission as a therapeutic tool. *Behav Sci Law, 18*(4), 459-477. https://doi.org/10.1002/1099-0798(2000)18:4<459::aid-bsl366>3.0.co;2-t

American Academy of Pediatrics Board of, D. (2020, Sep). Truth, Reconciliation, and Transformation: Continuing on the Path to Equity. *Pediatrics, 146*(3). https://doi.org/10.1542/peds.2020-019794

Avruch, K. (2010, Feb). Truth and reconciliation commissions: problems in transitional justice and the reconstruction of identity. *Transcult Psychiatry, 47*(1), 33-49. https://doi.org/10.1177/1363461510362043

Baines, E. (2010). Spirits and social reconstruction after mass violence: rethinking transitional justice. *Afr Aff (Lond), 109*(436), 409-430. https://doi.org/10.1093/afraf/adq023

Beckmann, J., Wenzel, T., Hautzinger, M., & Kizilhan, J. I. (2022). Training of psychotherapists in post-conflict regions: A Community case study in the Kurdistan Region of Iraq. *Front Psychiatry, 13*, 947903. https://doi.org/10.3389/fpsyt.2022.947903

Caparos, S., Rutembesa, E., Habimana, E., & Blanchette, I. (2020, Oct). The psychological correlates of transitional justice in Rwanda: A long-term assessment. *Psychol Trauma, 12*(7), 774-784. https://doi.org/10.1037/tra0000583

Cunningham, J. E. A., & Shapiro, C. M. (2018, Mar). Cognitive Behavioural Therapy for Insomnia (CBT-I) to treat depression: A systematic review. *J Psychosom Res, 106*, 1-12. \ https://doi.org/10.1016/j.jpsychores.2017.12.012

Frank, H. E., Becker-Haimes, E. M., & Kendall, P. C. (2020, Sep). Therapist training in evidence-based interventions for mental health: A systematic review of training approaches and outcomes. *Clin Psychol (New York), 27*(3). https://doi.org/10.1111/cpsp.12330

Gilmore, S. A. (2018). United Nations Security Council Resolution 2379. *International Legal Materials, 57*(5), 960-965. https://doi.org/10.1017/ilm.2018.41

Graybill, L. (2001). The contribution of the Truth and Reconciliation Commission toward the promotion of women's rights in South Africa. *Womens Stud Int Forum, 24*(1), 1-10. https://doi.org/10.1016/s0277-5395(00)00160-6

Iacopino, V., Haar, R. J., Heisler, M., Lin, J., Fincanci, S. K., Esdaile, C., Modvig, J., Sveaass, N., Nathanson, V. H., Melzer, N., & Cohen, J. (2022, Jul 16). Istanbul Protocol 2022 empowers health professionals to end torture. *Lancet, 400*(10347), 143-145. https://doi.org/10.1016/S0140-6736(22)00948-5

Johnson, C., AlRasheed, R., Gray, C., Triplett, N., Mbwayo, A., Weinhold, A., Whetten, K., & Dorsey, S. (2024, Jan-Dec). Uncovering determinants of perceived feasibility of TF-CBT through coincidence analysis. *Implement Res Pract, 5*, 26334895231220277. https://doi.org/10.1177/26334895231220277

Kananian, S., Starck, A., & Stangier, U. (2021, Nov). Cultural Adaptation of CBT for Afghan Refugees in Europe: A Retrospective Evaluation. *Clin Psychol Eur, 3*(Spec Issue), e5271. https://doi.org/10.32872/cpe.5271

Kaplan, S. (2014). *Social covenants and social contracts in transitions*. https://www.files.ethz.ch/isn/177459/59a4b4b0865e7aa4404f8ec04421b1e1.pdf

Kienzler, H. (2019a, Nov). Mental health in all policies in contexts of war and conflict. *Lancet Public Health, 4*(11), e547-e548. https://doi.org/10.1016/S2468-2667(19)30208-7

Kienzler, H. (2019b, Dec). Mental Health System Reform in Contexts of Humanitarian Emergencies: Toward a Theory of "Practice-Based Evidence". *Cult Med Psychiatry, 43*(4), 636-662. https://doi.org/10.1007/s11013-019-09641-w

Kirkpatrick, M. E., Dawley, A., & et al. (1949, Jan). Training for psychotherapy with special reference to nonmedical fields. *Am J Orthopsychiatry, 19*(1), 1-55. https://doi.org/10.1111/j.1939-0025.1949.tb06550.x

Kizilhan, J. I. (2014, Jun). Religious and cultural aspects of psychotherapy in Muslim patients from tradition-oriented societies. *Int Rev Psychiatry, 26*(3), 335-343. https://doi.org/10.3109/09540261.2014.899203

Kizilhan, J. I. (2017, Dec 28). Trauma and Pain in Family-Orientated Societies. *Int J Environ Res Public Health, 15*(1). https://doi.org/10.3390/ijerph15010044

Kizilhan, J. I., Berger, T., Sennhauser, L., & Wenzel, T. (2023). The psychological impact of genocide on the Yazidis. *Front Psychol, 14*, 1074283. https://doi.org/10.3389/fpsyg.2023.1074283

Kizilhan, J. I., Friedl, N., Neumann, J., & Traub, L. (2020, May 24). Potential trauma events and the psychological consequences for Yazidi women after ISIS captivity. *BMC Psychiatry, 20*(1), 256. https://doi.org/10.1186/s12888-020-02671-4

Kizilhan, J. I., & Neumann, J. (2020). The Significance of Justice in the Psychotherapeutic Treatment of Traumatized People After War and Crises. *Front Psychiatry, 11*, 540. https://doi.org/10.3389/fpsyt.2020.00540

Kizilhan, J. I., & Noll-Hussong, M. (2017, Dec 11). Individual, collective, and transgenerational traumatization in the Yazidi. *BMC Med, 15*(1), 198. https://doi.org/10.1186/s12916-017-0965-7

Kizilhan, J. I., & Wenzel, T. (2020, Nov-Dec). Positive psychotherapy in the treatment of traumatised Yezidi survivors of sexualised violence and genocide. *Int Rev Psychiatry, 32*(7-8), 594-605. https://doi.org/10.1080/09540261.2020.1809356

Koseoglu, Z. (2022). Launch of the revised version on the Istanbul Protocol. *Torture, 32*(3), 89. https://doi.org/10.7146/torture.v32i3.133934

Lin, C. Y., Meagher, K., Bricknell, M., Patel, P., El Achi, N., Kutluk, T., Harding, R., Kienzler, H., Giacaman, R., Mukherji, D., Shamieh, O., & Sullivan, R. (2023, Jun 14). The challenges of international collaboration in conflict and health research: experience from the Research for Health in Conflict-Middle East and North Africa (R4HC-MENA) partnership. *Confl Health, 17*(1), 29. https://doi.org/10.1186/s13031-023-00527-8

Lott, G. M. (1952, Jul). The training of non-medical cooperative psychotherapists by multiple psychotherapy. *Am J Psychother, 6*(3), 440-448. https://doi.org/10.1176/appi.psychotherapy.1952.6.3.440

Luchines, A. S. (1949, Apr). On training clinical psychologists in psychotherapy. *J Clin Psychol, 5*(2), 132-137. https://doi.org/10.1002/1097-4679(194904)5:2<132::aid-jclp2270050205>3.0.co;2-8

Madu, S. N., Baguma, P., Pritz, A., & World Council for Psychotherapy. (1998). *In quest for psychotherapy for modern Africa*. UNIN Press.

Marshall, C. (2022, Sep). The inter-agency standing committee (IASC) guidelines on mental health and psychosocial support (MHPSS) in emergency settings: a critique. *Int Rev Psychiatry, 34*(6), 604-612. https://doi.org/10.1080/09540261.2022.2147420

Mathias, K., Bunkley, N., Pillai, P., Ae-Ngibise, K. A., Kpobi, L., Taylor, D., Joag, K., Rawat, M., Hammoudeh, W., Mitwalli, S., Kagee, A., van

Rensburg, A., Bemme, D., Burgess, R. A., Jain, S., Kienzler, H., & Read, U. M. (2024). Inverting the deficit model in global mental health: An examination of strengths and assets of community mental health care in Ghana, India, Occupied Palestinian territories, and South Africa. *PLOS Glob Public Health, 4*(3), e0002575. https://doi.org/10.1371/journal.pgph.0002575

Matyas, D., Akhavan, P., Ashraph, S., & Barzani, B. (2020, 02/01). What Justice for the Yazidi Genocide?: Voices from Below. *Human Rights Quarterly, 42*, 1-47. https://doi.org/10.1353/hrq.2020.0000

Mayor, S. (2008, Aug 27). WHO calls for better living conditions to reduce health gap. *BMJ, 337*, a1451. https://doi.org/10.1136/bmj.a1451

McGibbon, E. (2019, Jan). Truth and reconciliation: Healthcare organizational leadership. *Healthc Manage Forum, 32*(1), 20-24. https://doi.org/10.1177/0840470418803379

Naeem, F., Latif, M., Mukhtar, F., Kim, Y. R., Li, W., Butt, M. G., Kumar, N., & Ng, R. (2021, Mar). Transcultural adaptation of cognitive behavioral therapy (CBT) in Asia. *Asia Pac Psychiatry, 13*(1), e12442. https://doi.org/10.1111/appy.12442

Nashwan, A. J., Osman, S. H., & Mohamedahmed, L. A. (2023, Jun). Violence in Sudan: A Looming Public Health Disaster. *Cureus, 15*(6), e40343. https://doi.org/10.7759/cureus.40343

Neumann, J. C., Berger, T., & Kizilhan, J. I. (2021, Nov 24). Development of a Questionnaire to Measure the Perceived Injustice of People Who Have Experienced Violence in War and Conflict Areas: Perceived Injustice Questionnaire (PIQ). *Int J Environ Res Public Health, 18*(23). https://doi.org/10.3390/ijerph182312357

Pasternack, S. A. (1977, Nov). The psychotherapy fee: an issue in residency training. *Dis Nerv Syst, 38*(11), 913-916. https://www.ncbi.nlm.nih.gov/pubmed/913226

Pham, P. N., Vinck, P., & Weinstein, H. M. (2010, Jan). Human rights, transitional justice, public health and social reconstruction. *Soc Sci Med, 70*(1), 98-105. https://doi.org/10.1016/j.socscimed.2009.09.039

Pinchuk, I., Yachnik, Y., Kopchak, O., Avetisyan, K., Gasparyan, K., Ghazaryan, G., Chkonia, E., Panteleeva, L., Guerrero, A., & Skokauskas, N. (2021, Apr 21). The Implementation of the WHO Mental Health Gap Intervention Guide (mhGAP-IG) in Ukraine, Armenia, Georgia and Kyrgyz Republic. *Int J Environ Res Public Health, 18*(9). https://doi.org/10.3390/ijerph18094391

Praptomojati, A., Icanervilia, A. V., Nauta, M. H., & Bouman, T. K. (2024, Feb). A systematic review of Culturally Adapted Cognitive Behavioral Therapy (CA-CBT) for anxiety disorders in Southeast Asia. *Asian J Psychiatr, 92*, 103896. https://doi.org/10.1016/j.ajp.2023.103896

Rennie, T. A. (1947, May). Psychotherapy for the general practitioner; a program for training; post-graduate education. *Am J Psychiatry, 103*(5), 653-660. https://doi.org/10.1176/ajp.103.5.653

Sewordor, E., Esnard, A. M., Sapat, A., & Schwartz, L. (2019, Apr). Challenges to mobilising resources for disaster recovery and reconstruction: perspectives of the Haitian diaspora. *Disasters, 43*(2), 336-354. https://doi.org/10.1111/disa.12318

Spenceley, S. (2016, Spring). Rising to the Challenge of the Truth and Reconciliation Commission. *Alta RN, 72*(1), 3. https://www.ncbi.nlm.nih.gov/pubmed/27290769

Swartz, L., & Drennan, G. (2000, Aug-Nov). The cultural construction of healing in the Truth and Reconciliation Commission: implications for mental health practice. *Ethn Health, 5*(3-4), 205-213. https://doi.org/10.1080/713667455

Wenzel T, A. R., Kizilhan J, Wittek TU (2023). Collecting Evidence and Testimonies of Severe Human Rights Violations – The Importance of the Mind. *ARCH Women Health Care 62*(2), 1-4. https://doi.org/10.31038/AWHC.2023621

Wenzel, T., Frewer, A., & Mirzaei, S. (2015). The DSM 5 and the Istanbul Protocol: Diagnosis of psychological sequels of torture. *Torture, 25*(1), 51-61. https://www.ncbi.nlm.nih.gov/pubmed/26021347

Wenzel, T., Kizilhan, J. I., Alksiri, R., Dorfler, D., Messerschmidt, E. J., & Chen, A. F. (2021, Aug 24). FGM and Restorative Justice-A Challenge for Developing Countries and for Refugee Women. *Int J Environ Res Public Health, 18*(17). https://doi.org/10.3390/ijerph18178913

Wilfley, D. E., Agras, W. S., Fitzsimmons-Craft, E. E., Bohon, C., Eichen, D. M., Welch, R. R., Jo, B., Raghavan, R., Proctor, E. K., & Wilson, G. T. (2020, Feb 1). Training Models for Implementing Evidence-Based Psychological Treatment: A Cluster-Randomized Trial in College Counseling Centers. *JAMA Psychiatry, 77*(2), 139-147. https://doi.org/10.1001/jamapsychiatry.2019.3483

CHAPTER 3

STRENGTHENING MENTAL HEALTH SERVICES IN CRISIS AREAS: BEYOND MHPSS APPROACHES

JAN ILHAN KIZILHAN

While community-oriented models of Mental Health and Psychosocial Support (MHPSS) have been instrumental in addressing mental health challenges arising from mass violence and conflict, some studies suggest that the immediate application of psychosocial interventions after disasters may not be the primary concern. This perspective aligns with the principles of psychological first aid (Meewisse et al., 2011; World Health Organization, 2011).

The primary focus should be on ensuring people feel safe and experience a reduction in anxiety after a disaster. Achieving this requires the provision of information, sufficient food, housing, access to medical care, and psychological first aid (see Table 3-1). The goal is to help individuals alleviate stress, achieve a state of calmness, and attain both psychological and physical comfort (Forbes et al., 2011).

Table 3-1 Interventions in the Aftermath of Disasters

Intervention	Target population	Examples of Interventions	Intervention conducted by
Finding people and protecting them from further threats	Most of the people who are affected	Professionals and any person who can help to protect them	Military Policy Community
Relocate to a safe place if possible	Most of the people who are affected	Put in a safe place (house, building, tent etc.)	Police Health Staff

Emergency first aid	Most of the people who are affected	Physical examination, first treatment of injuries	Physician Aid workers
Medical examination	Most of the people who are affected	Physical examination, outpatient or inpatient treatment	Physician
Psychological first aid	Most of the people who are affected	Restoring immediate safety, restoring contact with loved ones	All responders and aid workers
Initial psychological examination and diagnostics	For people with first psychological symptoms, like acute stress disorder (ADS)	Assessment of anxiety, seizures, state of shock, first depressive symptoms, sleeping disorder, nightmares, social isolation	Psychiatrist Psychotherapist Clinical Psychologist
Psychological examination and diagnostics after one month	People who meet the criteria for PTSD	Psychological screening and assessment, determination of the need for long-term psychotherapy	Psychiatrist Psychotherapist Clinical Psychologist
Skills for psychosocial recovery	People whose distress is sustained by bereavement or secondary stressors	Brief assessment of needs, problem-solving, social support	Healthcare practitioners and workers with expertise in implementing the required skills

Psychosocial interventions for medium- and long-term problems Outpatient and/or inpatient psychiatric treatment	People whose distress is sustained and associated with functional impairment	Culturally sensitive adapted Psychotrauma-Therapy	Staff of mental healthcare facilities: Psychiatrists, Psychotherapists, Clinical Psychologists, social workers specialized in trauma

Many of the temporary symptoms and discomfort that occur after a disaster can be addressed through MHPSS approaches. These approaches have been used in Iraq and have proved to be effective in reducing psychological symptomatology (Al-Khalisi, 2013). However, their effectiveness in preventing severe and enduring mental disorders, such as PTSD, is limited (Beckmann et al., 2022). The diagnosis and treatment of these disorders requires specialized personnel like psychiatrists or psychotherapists, which are often scarce in regions affected by ongoing conflicts and war. Therefore, it is imperative to establish academic structures which ensure continuous professional training in regions affected by ongoing conflicts and post-conflict difficulties, contributing to a sustainable solution for mental health challenges into the future. In response to this pressing need in Northern Iraq, the Duhok Project was launched, leading to the establishment of the Institute for Psychotherapy and Psychotraumatology. The next chapter provides an in-depth exploration of this essential initiative.

References

Al-Khalisi, N. (2013). The Iraqi medical brain drain: A cross-sectional study. *International Journal of Health Services*, *43*(2), 363-378. https://doi.org/10.2190/HS.43.2.j

Beckmann, J., Wenzel, T., Hautzinger, M., & Kizilhan, J. I. (2022). Training of psychotherapists in post-conflict regions: A Community case study in the Kurdistan Region of Iraq [Community Case Study]. *Frontiers in Psychiatry*, *13*. https://doi.org/10.3389/fpsyt.2022.947903

Forbes, D., Lewis, V., Varker, T., Phelps, A., O'Donnell, M., Wade, D. J., Ruzek, J. I., Watson, P., Bryant, R. A., & Creamer, M. (2011). Psychological first aid following trauma: Implementation and evaluation framework for high-risk organizations. *Psychiatry: Interpersonal & Biological Processes*, *74*(3), 224-239.

Meewisse, M. L., Olff, M., Kleber, R., Kitchiner, N. J., & Gersons, B. P. (2011). The course of mental health disorders after a disaster: Predictors and comorbidity. *Journal of Traumatic Stress*, *24*(4), 405-413.

World Health Organization. (2011). *Psychological first aid: Guide for field workers*. World Health Organization.

CHAPTER 4

HISTORY AND SOCIAL STRUCTURE OF MODERN IRAQ

JAN ILHAN KIZILHAN AND ANNA WEIGELT

This chapter provides a concise overview of Iraq's history since the outbreak of World War I, with a particular focus on its ethnic and religious diversity, as well as the Kurdish independence efforts in northern Iraq. This chapter serves as a contextual analysis, essential for laying the groundwork for culturally sensitive health initiatives, such as the Duhok project.

Iraq's History between World War I and the US Invasion

Iraq roughly corresponds to the ancient territory of Mesopotamia and translates from Greek as "the land between the two rivers," the Tigris and the Euphrates. Iraq is located between Kuwait and Saudi Arabia to the south, Jordan to the west, Syria to the north-west, Turkey to the north, and Iran is to the east (Seymour, 2004). It spans an area of 434,924 square kilometers, is divided into 18 governates, and has a population of 44,496,122 people as of 2022 (World Bank, 2022).

Amidst the outbreak of World War I, the alignment between the Ottoman Empire and Germany raised concerns for Britain, prompting a strategic interest in gaining control over Mesopotamia. This aim was rooted in the protection of communication routes and newly discovered oil fields situated in Kuwait, at the northern extent of the Gulf. The initial British military engagement was concentrated in Basra, located at the head of the Gulf, followed by a broader campaign to extend influence across the entire region that is now known as Iraq (Kirmanj, 2013).

A revolution in 1958 transformed the country from a monarchy under colonial rule into a republic. This republic sought to avoid the existing Cold War power dynamics and to promote autonomous national prosperity. Up until the late 1960s, authoritarian monarchs quickly changed positions of power, backed by different military forces (Hopwood et al., 1993). Despite the ensuing political turbulence, and a murky, bloody conflict with Iran in the early 1970s (Halliday, 1990), the economy made exceptional progress. For example, between 1973 and 1975, the nationalization of oil businesses caused a nearly fourfold increase in oil income (Kirmanj, 2013).

After winning the presidency in 1979, Saddam Hussein established a dictatorship which was characterized by extreme repression internally, and repeated wars externally. The eight-year Iran-Iraq War, in which Iraq targeted Iranians as well as Iraqi Kurds, left physical and psychological scars on the country (Al-Ameri, 2012; Ghanei et al., 2010).

Iraq's subsequent invasion of Kuwait in 1990 resulted in international isolation and the 1991 Gulf War (Warbrick, 1991). Sanctions, political unrest, and regime changes ensued, culminating in the 2003 US-led invasion, and the final demise of Saddam Hussein's dictatorship. These events significantly damaged the country's stability, economy, and social fabric (Bassil, 2012). The disastrous course set by the occupying power's, particularly the dissolution of the Iraqi army and the active promotion of ethno-confessional structures in the establishment of the new political system, played a significant role in the country's subsequent decent into a period of recurring civil war between Shiite and Sunni groups (Jabar, 2007).

Focus Box: Ethnic and Religious Fragmentation

Iraq's demographic composition is made up by a complex interplay of ethnic and religious backgrounds. Islam is the national religion; around 97 percent of the population follows various types of Islam, while the remaining 3 percent is made up of a mix of Christians, Yazidis, Mandaeans, and Jews. Shia Arabs make up the majority of the ethnic background of Iraq (55% of the total Iraqi population), followed by Sunni Arabs (25% of the total population), and Kurds (20% of the population). Shiite communities are most prominent in the southern regions, Sunni Muslims predominantly reside in the midwestern and northwestern territories, and the Kurds in the elevated areas in the northeast (European Union Agency for Asylum, 2022; Kirmanj, 2013).

Though the war on terrorism has caused significant disruption in Iraq in recent years, the most important aspect of the country's dilemma is the ongoing conflicts and disagreements between Iraq's ethnic and religious groups regarding the nature, structure, and character of the state. The most serious challenge for the Iraqi people is ensuring the constitutional and institutional recognition and respect of the diverse cultural and national characteristics of Iraq's many communities.

Developments Since the War against ISIS

The formation of the Islamic State of Iraq and Syria (ISIS) in the mid-2010s, and the subsequent war in Iraq against ISIS between 2013 and 2017, was another defining episode in contemporary Iraq's history. ISIS rose to popularity in the aftermath of the US-led invasion of Iraq in 2003, driven by a power vacuum, sectarian tensions, and the disenfranchisement of some sectors of the population (Alaaldin, 2018).

In 2014, ISIS seized large areas of Iraqi land, including crucial cities like Mosul (Chulov, 2014). The group's brutal tactics, ideological fervor, and online propaganda drew international attention and condemnation (Beccaro, 2018; Mitts et al., 2022). The Iraqi government, in collaboration with a coalition of regional and global partners, mounted a strong counter-offensive to push back against ISIS (Glenn et al., 2019). ISIS progressively lost control of Iraq during several years of harsh struggle, including military battles, humanitarian disasters, and the displacement of millions (Coker & Hassan, 2017). Though militarily degraded, ISIS's influence on Iraq's culture, economy, and politics remains profound, highlighting difficulties in post-conflict stability and reconciliation.

Across Iraq's recent turbulent history, the Kurdish desire for self-governance further complicated the geopolitical situation. Although the Kurds have long aspired to establish their own nation state, this aspiration gained renewed momentum during the world wars, which resulted in the dispersal of the Kurds across several nations.

It wasn't until the 1990s that the Kurds made significant headway toward independence. Following the First Gulf War, the international community imposed a no-fly zone over northern Iraq, thereby providing the Kurds a degree of autonomy while Western forces protected them (Sherwani, 2021).

After Saddam Hussein's dictatorship fell in 2003, this autonomy gained traction. In 2005, the Kurdistan Region of Iraq (KRI) was acknowledged as an autonomous region (within Iraq) in the new Iraqi constitution. The Kurdistan Regional Government (KRG) was consequently formed (Kurdistan Regional Government, 2023).

Attempts to entirely split from Iraq have elicited conflicting international reactions. The Kurdistan Region's 2017 independence referendum, which saw an overwhelming majority vote in favor of separation (Chulov, 2017; O'Driscoll & Baser, 2019), was opposed by the Iraqi government, neighboring nations, and global powers. As a result, the push for full independence has not materialized, and negotiations between the KRG and the central Iraqi government are still ongoing.

Iraq's political environment is still volatile today. The new government elected in October 2021 will be tasked with initiating a number of structural reforms, including reducing economic reliance on oil exports, resolving social tensions and ethno-religious conflicts, preventing corruption and nepotism, ensuring basic services for the population, and resolving conflicts over resources and territorial claims between the central government and the KRI (Fazil & Tartir, 2023).

References

Al-Ameri, M. H. I. (2012). Effectiveness of a psychosocial rehabilitation programme for Iraqi repatriated prisoners of the Iran-Iraq War, 1980-1988. Liverpool John Moores University (United Kingdom).

Alaaldin, R. (2018). Sectarianism, governance, and Iraq's future. Brookings Doha Center Analysis Paper, 24.

Bassil, Y. (2012). The 2003 Iraq war: operations, causes, and consequences. Journal of Humanities and Social Science, 4(5), 29-47.

Beccaro, A. (2018). Modern irregular warfare: The ISIS case study. Small Wars & Insurgencies, 29(2), 207-228.

Chulov, M. (2014). ISIS insurgents seize control of Iraqi city of Mosul. The Guardian, 10, 2014.

Chulov, M. (2017). More than 92% of voters in Iraqi Kurdistan back independence. The Guardian, 28.

Coker, M., & Hassan, F. (2017). Iraq Prime Minister declares victory over ISIS. New York Times, 9.

European Union Agency for Asylum. (2022). Country Guidance: Iraq. Publications Office of the European Union. https://books.google.de/books?id=9KK0zwEACAAJ

Fazil, S., & Tartir, A. (2023). Iraq in 2023: Challenges and prospects for peace and human security. Stockholm International Peace Research Institute. Retrieved 01.08.23 from
\ https://www.sipri.org/commentary/topical-backgrounder/2023/iraq-2023-challenges-and-prospects-peace-and-human-security

Ghanei, M., Naderi, M., Kosar, A. M., Harandi, A. A., Hopkinson, N. S., & Poursaleh, Z. (2010). Long-term pulmonary complications of chemical warfare agent exposure in Iraqi Kurdish civilians. Inhalation Toxicology, 22(9), 719-724. https://doi.org/10.3109/08958371003686016

Glenn, C., Rowan, M., Caves, J., & Nada, G. (2019). Timeline: The rise, spread, and fall of the Islamic State. Wilson Center. Retrieved 21.08.23 from https://www.wilsoncenter.org/article/timeline-the-rise-spread-and-fall-the-islamic-state

Halliday, F. (1990). Iraq and its neighbours: the cycles of insecurity. The World Today, 46(6), 104-106.

Hopwood, D., Ishow, H., & Koszinowski, T. (1993). Iraq: power and society (Vol. 10). Ithaca Press (GB).

Ireland, P. W. (2013). Iraq: A study in political development. Routledge.

Jabar, F. A. (2007). Iraq Four Years after the US-Led Invasion: Assessing the Crisis and Searching for A Way Forward.‖ Policy Outlook. In: CARNEGIE Endowment for International Peace.

Kirmanj, S. (2013). Identity and Nation in Iraq. Lynne Rienner Publishers. https://doi.org/doi:10.1515/9781626370791

Kurdistan Regional Government. (2023). Facts & Figures. Kurdistan Regional Government. Retrieved 22.08.23 from https://gov.krd/boi-en/why-kurdistan/region/facts-figures/

Mitts, T., Phillips, G., & Walter, B. F. (2022). Studying the impact of ISIS propaganda campaigns. The Journal of Politics, 84(2), 1220-1225.

O'Driscoll, D., & Baser, B. (2019). Independence referendums and nationalist rhetoric: the Kurdistan Region of Iraq. Third World Quarterly, 40(11), 2016-2034.

Seymour, M. (2004). Ancient Mesopotamia and modern Iraq in the British press, 1980–2003. Current Anthropology, 45(3), 351-368.

Sherwani, H. (2021). No fly zone: the pillar of Iraqi Kurds' survival. Kurdistan 24. Retrieved 21.08.23 from https://www.kurdistan24.net/en/story/24221-No-fly-zone:-the-pillar-of-Iraqi-Kurds%E2%80%99-survival

Warbrick, C. (1991). The Invasion of Kuwait by Iraq. The International and Comparative Law Quarterly, 40(2), 482-492. http://www.jstor.org/stable/759738

World Bank. (2022). Population, total - Iraq. The World Bank Group. Retrieved 19.08.23 from https://data.worldbank.org/indicator/SP.POP.TOTL?locations=IQ&most_recent_value_desc=true

CHAPTER 5

DEVELOPMENT OF THE IRAQI HEALTH SYSTEM

JAN ILHAN KIZILHAN AND ANNA WEIGELT

This chapter provides an overview of the development of the Iraqi and northern Iraqi healthcare systems, highlighting both the available resources and the existing gaps and challenges. This chapter should be viewed as part of a needs assessment, which preceded the Duhok project and is a critical step in the implementation of healthcare initiatives, standing alongside the analysis of historical and social contexts.

Evolution from 1950s to Modern Day

The development of the Iraqi health system is closely tied to the wars and conflicts that Iraq has both initiated and experienced. With the establishment of the Iraqi Ministry of Health (MoH) in 1952, the country worked steadily to establish a highly centralized, hospital-oriented health care system (Alwan, 2004; World Health Organization, 2006). During the 1970s and 1980s, substantial revenue from thriving oil production enabled the government to fully subsidize free health care, supported by a high-quality medical education system. At the time, well-trained medical professionals, who often received additional specialty training abroad (Al Hilfi et al., 2013), provided excellent health care across 172 hospitals and 1200 primary health-care clinics . As a result, by 1980, Iraq ranked not only among the strongest economies in the Middle East but also had one of the best healthcare systems in the region (Henderson & United States Institute of, 2005).

After Saddam Hussein came to power in 1979, Iraq's health care system began to deteriorate. While the Iran-Iraq war (1980-1988) led to the first substantial funding cuts to public services, the invasion of Kuwait in 1990 left the country with high levels of debt and little resources to allocate towards the health sector. Scholarships for physicians to pursue training abroad were reduced and human resources were depleted, as many doctors were required to join the military (Al Hilfi et al., 2013; Al-Bayan

Center for Planning and Studies, 2018). The lack of medical resources, training opportunities, and dangerous working environments were accompanied by a system of repression and violence, leading to the first wave of medical personnel fleeing the country (Sadik & Al-Jadiry, 2006; Younis & Khunda, 2020).

The situation worsened with the start of the Gulf War in 1991, leading to the destruction of Iraq's entire infrastructure, including electricity, roads, bridges, and telecommunications. Extensive UN-sanctions were also introduced for thirteen years (Younis & Khunda, 2020). As a result of sanctions, export restrictions, and the destruction of numerous oil wells, essential medications were in short supply and the Iraqi government had to reduce its budget for public health by 90% (IRFAD, 2014; Kapp, 2003; Zarocostas, 2007). Additionally, in the face of the threat of espionage, kidnapping, intimidation, travel restrictions, and a lack of resources and education, a second wave of health care professionals had to flee the country (Humphreys & Sadik, 2006).

In 2003, the Iraqi health system suffered further setbacks as a result of the US-led invasion and the ensuing political, economic, and security disruption. The invasion caused more damage and enabled looting of medical facilities, leading to significant losses of equipment and pharmaceutical supplies (Aziz, 2003; Kapp, 2003). After 2003, the Ministry of Health made valuable efforts to improve the health system by focusing on mental health and collaborating with individuals from Europe, Scandinavia, and the United States. Together, they worked on restoring the health system through conferences and training programs (Humphreys & Sadik, 2006). The Ministry also outlined plans to shift to a primary healthcare delivery system that was more decentralized and called for the establishment of a private sector to improve secondary and tertiary care (Ministry of Planning, 2010).

The violent rise of ISIS in 2014, and the accompanying fights to recapture Iraqi land between 2014 and 2017, further harmed the healthcare system, which had only begun to improve. Due to the intense fighting, a flood of families traumatized and injured from the war, had to seek shelter in refugee camps where sanitary conditions and medical care were inadequate. In areas controlled by ISIS, the situation was worse. Besides reserving specialized care and medications just for militants and their families, the terrorists denied medical help to anyone who was not directly connected to the group. Despite the militants' defeat, and the return of over 3.7 million Iraqis to their homes, the country's dire medical conditions have not significantly improved. This is due to the fact that nearly every hospital was destroyed in areas that ISIS once controlled. The destruction was frequently the result of militants exploiting hospitals as bases, which led to military strikes on the facilities (Henderson & United States Institute of, 2005).

The Current Health System

Infrastructure

The organizational framework of the existing Iraqi healthcare system has remained widely unchanged since the 1970s. It is divided into two primary levels: (1) the Federal Ministry of Health and Environment conducts the central planning and oversees 19 provincial health departments (one in each province and two in Baghdad), while (2) the Directorates of Health run the governorates on a local level. Together, they are responsible for 118 health districts, with each district serving 200,000-300,000 people (Finnish Immigration Service, 2019; World Health Organization, 2006). A network of hospitals and primary healthcare centers (PHCCs) deliver health services in the public sector. Preventive and basic healthcare services are provided by PHCCs. Hospitals receive referrals from PHCCs for patients who need specialized secondary and tertiary treatment. However, due to inequitable distribution, many Iraqis do not have easy access to hospitals (Cetorelli & Shabila, 2014; Godichet & Ghanem, 2004; Henderson & United States Institute of, 2005). Private hospitals also provide secondary and tertiary care; however, given there are no well-established health insurance programs in the country, private health care is paid out-of-pocket and is unfortunately well beyond the means of many Iraqis. Moreover, despite private hospitals being granted licenses by the Ministry of Health, they are largely unregulated by the national health oversight (Al Hilfi et al., 2013).

Resources

In 2022, a network of 281 public hospitals and 2,765 PHCCs provided low-cost services. The number of people served by each PHCC ranged between 10,000 and 45,000 persons (United Nations Iraq, 2022; World Health Organization, 2023). Hospital capacity in Iraq averages 1.3 beds per 1,000 people, and there are fewer than 800 intensive care unit (ICU) beds nationwide (Duran & Menon, 2020; World Bank). These figures demonstrate how few resources are available to meet the population's healthcare needs. There is also a scarcity of healthcare experts in Iraq. In 2020, there were 23.87 nurses per 10,000 people, compared to 9.66 medical doctors. Except for Iran, where the number of nurses was equivalent, these numbers of healthcare experts are lower than all of Iraq's neighboring nations. As a result, more than half of PHCCs have only one doctor on staff, with nurses and other healthcare personnel handling the rest of the work (World Health Organization, 2023).

The shortage of healthcare staff has an impact on mental health services as well. The World Health Organization (WHO) estimates that there are only 0.5 psychiatrists, 1.1 mental health nurses, 0.2 psychologists, and 0.05 social workers for every 100,000 Iraqis (World Health Organization, 2020). Another major source of concern is the high occurrence of dual practice among professionals in Iraq. Specifically, many doctors hold full-time positions with the Ministry of Health, while also working in the private sector. As a result, conflicts of interest may occur, which has the potential to affect how effectively and fairly healthcare is provided (Al Janabi & Chung, 2022). Tribes and militias are two additional issues that frequently drive medical professionals to seek out new lives, whether abroad or in another industry. Tribal people are said to seek vengeance on doctors when a tribal member dies, even if the doctor has done everything possible to save the patient. On the other hand, militias have been known to demand special treatment, even forcing doctors to abandon their existing patients in order to treat them (Bradley, 2016).

As previously stated, health insurance is not widely available in Iraq. While it is not commonly provided to the general public, it is often provided to employees in particular industries, such as financial services. This lack of comprehensive health insurance coverage places a financial burden on individuals and may hinder their access to necessary healthcare services (Finnish Immigration Service, 2019). Additionally, spending on the healthcare system in Iraq has dropped over time and remains relatively low compared to other Middle Eastern countries with comparable GDPs. In 2010, health accounted for around 8.4% of Iraq's GDP (USD 82.2 billion). By 2019, however, this percentage had dropped to 4.5% of Iraq's GDP, which had now risen to USD 110.83 billion. Furthermore, the use of public funds to support health services in the public sector has reduced in recent years (Al Hilfi et al., 2013; Al-Jumaili et al., 2021).

Access and Distribution

Access to healthcare also remains a major issue in Iraq. Only 40% of Iraqis are believed to have access to referral services, and it is estimated that 5.5 million Iraqis lack any access to medical care (Cetorelli & Shabila, 2014; UNOCHA, 2018). This is primarily due to a lack of funds and an uneven distribution of medical facilities and personnel (Cetorelli &

Shabila, 2014). The problem is exacerbated by the concentration of healthcare facilities and specialists in Baghdad, which makes it more difficult for people living outside the capital to access treatment (World Health Organization, 2024). In general, healthcare provider availability differs between rural and urban areas. Access to doctors is often better in metropolitan regions, whereas medical assistants provide most of healthcare in rural areas (Cetorelli & Shabila, 2014). Iraq's healthcare delivery faces certain challenges that additionally impact accessibility and connectivity. For example, unpaved roads and a lack of ambulances can make it difficult to get to health care facilities in remote locations. A family's average commute to the nearest PHCC takes more than 20 minutes, and in rural areas, this time can exceed up to 32 minutes (Al Hilfi, 2014).

Training and Education in General Medicine and Healthcare

Access to healthcare in Iraq is further hampered by a scarcity of drugs and qualified medical workers. Many senior doctors and consultants in Iraq were trained in Europe, but they were unable to retain contact with the global medical community due to sanctions. As a result, they continue to use outdated tools and procedures, which can impede the adoption of cutting-edge medical innovations (Aziz, 2003).

Mental Health Care

The mental health sector is overseen by the High Commission for Mental Health, an inter-administrative agency responsible for strategic planning and policy development in mental health care. It follows a three-tier system. Primary mental health care is provided in PHCCs, while secondary and tertiary mental health care is almost only available in larger hospitals with teaching responsibilities. This means that many individuals seeking outpatient care must rely on hospitals instead of primary-level services. Efforts are being made to shift the focus from a reliance on secondary and tertiary health care, towards community-oriented outpatient care. However, this requires significant investment in the development of secondary care facilities. Local initiatives are underway to establish day centers that can provide outpatient services, serving as a transition phase from inpatient care back to the community (Finnish Immigration Service, 2019).

There are 34 clinics across the country that specialize in providing mental health care (Finnish Immigration Service, 2019). However, Iraq barely has 400 psychiatrists, with only 100 to 200 of them working in the public sector. It is estimated that 5,000 psychiatrists are currently needed in Iraq, highlighting the significant scarcity of mental health experts. In some governorates, there is only one psychiatrist to service the entire population (Finnish Immigration Service, 2019).

By 2019, Iraq had four hospitals dedicated to specialist psychiatric care. Two of these facilities, Al Rashad and Ibn Rushd, are in Baghdad, while the other two hospitals are in Sulaymaniyah (which is in Iraqi Kurdistan) and Diwaniya (which is in the governorate of Al-Qadisiyah) (Finnish Immigration Service, 2019).

Iraq has made more financial investments in the treatment of physical health disorders, than in the treatment of mental health difficulties. As such, the mental health care system has gaps in the education and training of mental health specialists (Finnish Immigration Service, 2019). Psychologists and social workers are frequently unable to provide evidence-based therapy due to a lack of a clinical component in their curriculum. Furthermore, specialist education programs are in short supply. In 2021, there was only one university in Iraq offering a master's degree program in clinical psychology, and clinical social work programs did not exist (Koya University, 2017; Murakami & Akilova, 2022).

The utilization of psychological expertise in the public sector is also limited, as individuals trained as psychologists are typically employed in non-healthcare positions, such as school psychologists. Similarly, the private sector prioritizes psychiatrists over psychologists, further restricting access to psychological services in mental health care. Iraqi medical school graduates frequently decide against specializing in psychiatry because of the persistent stigma associated with mental health conditions. In addition, some psychiatrists lack the necessary knowledge and experience to treat a wide range of mental disorders, or manage a heavy patient caseload (Finnish Immigration Service, 2019).

Another significant challenge facing the mental health sector in Iraq is the high prevalence of secondary traumatic stress among mental health professionals, a condition arising from prolonged exposure to trauma experienced by others. A recent study among Iraqi psychotherapists revealed that nearly half (44.4%) experienced secondary traumatization (Kizilhan, 2020). Factors contributing to this high prevalence of secondary traumatization are complex and multifaceted. For example, many mental health professionals have personal trauma histories (44%) and a history of displacement (18.5%). Additionally, Kizilhan (2020) indicated that 30% of the female psychologists in their study reported that they were still directly affected by ISIS conflicts, as their husbands were fighting as Kurdish Peshmerga at the border with Syria. The struggle for recognition, poor remuneration, and the feeling of being inadequately qualified, further contribute to the situation. Additional risk factors include challenging working conditions in refugee camps, poor therapy environments, and inadequate collaboration with physicians (Kizilhan, 2020).

Iraq also lacks expertise in treating post-traumatic stress disorder (PTSD) and other illnesses brought on by trauma or conflict (Al-Bayan Center for Planning and Studies, 2018). However, there is acknowledgement of the potential benefits of innovative therapeutic approaches. Countries like Finland, known for their advancements in therapies such as music and art therapy, are highly regarded in Iraq for their success in stress management. Despite this, medication remains the primary method of treating mental health problems (Finnish Immigration Service, 2019).

Development of the Health System in Northern Iraq

In 1992, the Kurdistan Regional Government (KRG) in northern Iraq formed its own regional Ministry of Health, employing the same structure and management method as Baghdad. The KRG's health system has suffered comparable issues to Iraq's health system throughout the years (Karadaghi & Willott, 2015).

Difficulties and Challenges

Poor governance, corruption, and resource mismanagement have hindered the advancement of the KRG's health system (Tawfik-Shukor & Khoshnaw, 2010). Inadequate health education, limited medical research, and the limited influence of professional associations on the health system or private sector, are structural weaknesses which have led to a considerable number of medical graduates departing the region each year to work overseas.

In 2014, four interconnected crises further weakened the health care system: (1) a security crisis caused by the war with ISIS; (2) an economic crisis associated with a political impasse with the Iraqi national government; (3) an internal political crisis in the Kurdistan Region over resource control; and (4) a humanitarian crisis driven by millions of displaced people from central/southern Iraq and Syria (Abdallah et al., 2015; Middle East Research Institute, 2015; Ministry of Interior Joint Crisis Coordination Center; Pring, 2015).

Between January 2014 and May 2016, over 3.3 million individuals were displaced within Iraq. The majority of these internally displaced persons (IDPs) found refuge within the Kurdistan Region of Iraq (KRI). At the same time, the country had to deal with a massive influx of Syrian refugees, who fled their homeland in waves between August 2013 and late 2014. More than 244,000 refugees had fled to the KRI in 2015 (United Nations High Commissioner for Refugees, 2014). Tent settlements for refugees, which initially acted as emergency shelters, morphed into expansive slums as a result of continued displacement, with women and girls becoming vulnerable to gender-based violence. Several of Iraq's largest cities ended up taking in more IDPs, exceeding the number of people in their original populations, and putting tremendous strain on the host communities and the primary healthcare system. Overcrowded tent settlements exacerbated the stressful climate, further limiting healthcare access and quality (UN Habitat, 2024).

Despite substantial victories against ISIS in 2017, conditions for refugees in the KRI area rapidly deteriorated when the Iraqi Kurdistan referendum was held on September 25th, 2017. The KRI voted for independence from the Iraqi central government on that day. The referendum sparked tensions between the Kurdistan Regional Government and the Iraqi central government, as the Iraqi central government viewed the referendum as illegal and disruptive for the area. Baghdad responded to the referendum by taking a number of steps to seize control of the Kurdistan Region. Military actions included repossessing regions controlled by Kurdish troops during the war against ISIS, as well as barring international aircraft and trade across the Kurdistan Region's borders (Wörmer & Lamberty, 2018). Camp residents received sporadic food assistance, while those living in cities encountered additional burdens such as soaring living costs, medical fees, and a scarcity of job opportunities. For medical care, refugee camps relied on understaffed dispensaries that often lacked crucial medications. Outside of the camps, challenges intensified as a lack of health insurance limited access to medical services, forcing reliance on medical check-ups at public clinics and hospitals (Syrian Civic Platform, 2018).

The already high prevalence of mental disorders was exacerbated the humanitarian crisis. A study among Syrian refugees in the KRI found that 54.3% met DSM-5 PTSD symptom criteria, while 59.8% met major depressive disorder diagnostic criteria (Mahmood et al., 2022). Similarly, an investigation focused on IDPs situated in the Duhok province reported a prevalence rate of 29.1% for PTSD among females and 31.9% among their male counterparts (Taha & Sijbrandij, 2021). These trends were most pronounced among individuals who had undergone prolonged and repetitive exposure to traumatic events. Among Yazidi IDPs living in a refugee camp within the KRI, a striking 79% reported experiencing PTSD symptoms (Al Shawi & Hassen, 2022). When focusing on Yazidi women who had survived the 2014 genocide and endured captivity by ISIS, the prevalence was even more staggering, with 97.9% displaying symptoms indicative of PTSD and 88.1% indicative of major depression (Kizilhan et al., 2020).

In 2022, Iraq still was home to a substantial population of approximately 1.2 million IDPs and 273,716 refugees from Syria, Iran, and Palestine. Around 40% of refugees were living in camp settings, while the rest were residing in informal settings among the host populations (Kurdistan Regional Government, 2023a; UNHCR, 2023a, 2023b). Between 2014 and 2022, the KRI, encompassing a population of approximately 5.2 million individuals (Kurdistan Regional Government, 2024), provided sanctuary to an astounding six million IDPs and refugees (UNHCR, 2022). Despite the high degree of acceptance by both authorities and the local population, as well as ongoing efforts to stabilize the humanitarian situation in the region through various initiatives, a significant number of refugees continue to face hurdles related to security threats, protection concerns, and a lack of opportunities for integration. These obstacles lead to restricted livelihood options, limited financial means during displacement and upon return home, and the absence of crucial civil documentation. Furthermore, difficulties in accessing adequate healthcare persist (UNHCR, 2022, 2023a). In 2022, 86% of Syrian refugees based in camps experienced food insecurity (United Nations, 2022).

Insufficient availability and quality of services, as well as medical equipment, led the public sector to reorient towards primary health care (Shabila et al., 2010). Unfortunately, the quantity and distribution of physician-staffed PHCCs never reached global standards, with less than 30% of PHCCs having at least one physician. Up until today, the services provided by various facilities are not consistent, and referrals are not effectively coordinated. The availability and quality of primary care varies, and there is a lack of systematic measurement and training in quality improvement strategies. Physicians are dispersed unevenly, overworked, and predominantly devoted to private practice, whereas nurses are underutilized and undertrained. Health information systems are undervalued, with inefficient data collection and processing, limited use of computer technologies, and insufficient patient recording. The finance structure is primarily reliant on government funds, with little incentive for efficiency, and there is barely any private insurance (Shabila et al., 2010).

Strengths in Human Resources and Facilities

Although the KRI's health-care system still faces numerous challenges, it has consistently provided better medical care than the rest of Iraq. More stable political conditions and reliable security make it more secure than the rest of Iraq, and therefore more appealing to medical professionals from the southern and central parts of the country (Al Hilfi et al., 2013; Price, 2018). Despite the rate of population growth being similar in KRI and central/southern Iraq, the number of PHCCs per 100,000 people increased at different rates in these areas between 2003 and 2012. In Kurdistan, there was an average increase of 4.3 PHCCs per 100,000 people, compared to an increase of only 1.4 PHCCs per 100,000 people in Iraq. Furthermore, in 2012, there were 0.4 to 0.8 public hospitals per 100,000 people in the central and southern governorates, compared to 1.1 to 1.7 in the Kurdish governorates (Cetorelli & Shabila, 2014). These large disparities in the number of health-care facilities between the KRI and the rest of Iraq continue to this day (Al Janabi & Chung, 2022).

The improvement in health infrastructure may be attributed mostly to the Oil for Food Program (OFFP). After five years of stringent international sanctions, the UN Security Council approved the OFFP, allowing Iraq to spend its oil profits for humanitarian reasons (United Nations Office of the Iraq Programme Oil-for-Food, 2004a). In Kurdistan, the program was supervised directly by UN agencies, while the remainder of the nation was overseen by the Iraqi government. In contrast to little government expenditure for health infrastructure in central and southern Iraq, UNICEF and UN-Habitat constructed a large number of new health facilities, mostly PHCCs, in Kurdistan (United Nations Office of the Iraq Programme Oil-for-Food, 2004b). Since 2007, the Kurdistan regional administration has also adopted a liberal investment approach that has drawn more domestic and international investors to a variety of sectors, including health care (Kurdistan Regional Government, 2021).

The medical education system in the KRI is largely based on the standard Iraqi curriculum, following the traditional six-year British model (Husni et al., 2006). However, in contrast to central and southern Iraq, numerous initiatives have been implemented to raise educational standards (Saleh et al., 2015). For example, the Ministry of Higher Education in the KRG was able to substantially promote continuous medical education and professional growth through a $100 million USD initiative known as the "Human Capacity Development Program" (HCDP). This program provided assistance to postgraduate MSc and PhD programs at medical institutions in the KRI region (Kok et al., 2014). Additionally, the Kurdistan Board of Medical specializations (KBMS) was established in 2009 in response to the need to improve healthcare services. The KBMS is a medical sciences education and training organization. Its major purpose is to certify doctors as experts in numerous medical specialties, including psychiatry, and to advance their professional standing in alignment with the most recent global standards (Kurdistan Board of Medical Specialities, 2018).

Mental Health Care

Like central/southern Iraq, the KRI's mental health sector is characterized by stigma, negative attitudes towards mental illness and help-seeking behaviors, insufficient mental health education, and the absence of formal reviews of existing psychiatric services (Al-Salihy & Rahim, 2013; Bolton, 2013). This is partially due to the lack of clinical psychology or psychotherapy expertise in healthcare education, academic institutions, and medical schools. Psychotherapists are not distinguished from other types of healthcare professionals, like social workers or counselors. Psychotherapy is not governed by legislation, and little is known about the profession of a psychotherapist in the KRI (Beckmann et al., 2022; Halaj & Huppert, 2017).

However, initiatives to enhance psychiatric treatment and mental health services in the KRI have increased recently. This is due to the humanitarian crisis, which has prompted a substantial influx of international NGOs and other key players engaged in development-oriented humanitarian emergency responses. Notable organizations include the World Health Organization (WHO), the UN Refugee Agency (UNHCR), the International Organization for Migration (ION), Médecins du Monde (MDM), and International Medical Corps (IMC) (Böge et al., 2022; Shukor et al., 2017; World Health Organization, 2016a). By the beginning of 2023, the Kurdistan Region had officially registered 4737 NGOs. Of these organizations, 587 were Iraqi or international, while 3967 were Kurdish (Kurdistan Regional Government, 2023b).

Due to a shortage of specialized professionals, these organizations typically use the Inter-Agency Standing Committee (IASC) pyramid of interventions model. This model allows less specialized practitioners to provide Mental Health and Psychosocial Support (MHPSS) services, while concurrently offering training and supervision to fill gaps in MHPSS practitioners' expertise (Murakami & Akilova, 2022). While MHPSS teams usually comprise of psychologists, psychiatrists, and community workers, in the camps throughout the Duhok governorate community-based MHPSS is mostly provided by community workers who are primarily refugees themselves (Ali & Ari, 2021). Additionally, task-shifting strategies are used in these settings, including training non-specialized healthcare providers in

MHPSS methods and incorporating mental health treatment into basic healthcare (Bolton, 2019).

International players now exert a significant amount of influence and assistance in northern Iraq. In 2021, the WHO was able to deliver 10,521 MHPSS consultations, 270,133 PHCC consultations, and 5,828 specialized service referrals. A training program was also implemented to address rising suicide rates. Additionally, mental health experts and health care workers received training on referrals for gender-based violence victims, clinical management of rape, and psychosocial support for survivors (World Health Organization. Regional Office for the Eastern, 2022). In 2022, the International Organization for Migration provided 79,619 services and focused on creating programs to address the MHPSS needs of IDPs returning to their home countries. These programs aimed to prevent suicide and support the Yazidi community during the process of exhumation and reburial of genocide victims (IOM Iraq, 2023; Murakami & Akilova, 2022).

Focus Box: NGOs Active in the KRI

Problem Management+ (PM+), World Health Organization (WHO)

Recognizing the potential of community workers, and the urgent need for psychotherapy, a movement towards low-intensity psychological therapies, conducted by experienced non-specialists, gained traction (Collins et al., 2011). One example is Problem Management Plus (PM+), which was developed by the WHO to address common mental health concerns in adults, as well as practical obstacles such as unemployment (World Health Organization, 2016b). After making adjustments for Syrian refugees (Akhtar et al., 2020), UNHCR Iraq adapted PM+ into Badini Kurdish, the language spoken by Syrian Kurds in the Duhok region. In January 2020, the refugee MHPSS community workers who were supporting Duhok's four main refugee camps received PM+ training. The training sessions were highly interactive, with community workers suggesting contextual refinements. Trainees responded positively to the training, reporting personal and familial benefits beyond their roles, like increased empowerment and better social stress management (Ali & Ari, 2021). Subsequent research has demonstrated the efficacy of PM+ training in Iraq (Musotsi et al., 2022).

Free Yezidi Foundation (FYF)

The Free Yezidi Foundation (FYF) has a women's center in Iraq's Duhok region, which provides assistance to women in the Khanke IDP camp, including former ISIS captives. Their MHPSS program includes stabilization strategies like group EMDR therapy and trauma treatment approaches like psychoeducation, following IASC recommendations. Emotional recovery is aided through therapeutic interventions on an individual, group, and communal level, as well as by creative and physical activities. Service users who have received basic counseling training perform psychological first and second aid, while workshops raise trauma awareness (Womersley & Arikut-Treece, 2019).

Jiyan Foundation

The Jiyan Foundation stands at the forefront in the northern Kurdistan Region of Iraq and is committed to providing free mental health services. It achieves this by enlisting non-specialist psychotherapists who are trained in cognitive-behavioral therapies for PTSD, specific phobias, depression, and anxiety. Upon joining Jiyan, individuals holding a psychology bachelor's degree from Iraq or Kurdistan undertake a comprehensive 7-week psychotraumatology program, which is spread over a 2-year practical period. During this time, participants engage in hands-on practical work, applying their knowledge in real-world settings while simultaneously continuing their theoretical training. This training enables therapists to incorporate new knowledge into their client interactions, under the supervision of local Kurdish psychotherapists. Additionally, the formation of peer supervision groups brings trainees together to collectively complete assignments, enact role-play scenarios, and delve into the implementation of therapy techniques with clients. The program concludes with a written test based on an analysis of two treatment cases. A recent exploratory study showed that displaced individuals seeking therapy from psychotherapists trained at the Jiyan Foundation-experienced clinically significant reductions in both PTSD and depression symptoms (Blackwell et al., 2022).

Limitations of MHPSS Approaches

MHPSS approaches can be used to successfully treat a wide range of transient symptoms and discomforts that appear after a stressful event (Mukdarut et al., 2019). Taskshifting which refers to the delegation of tasks from specialized professionals to less specialized workers to make more efficient use of the available workforce, has been successfully used in Iraq and has been shown to reduce psychological symptomatology (Al-Khalisi, 2013; Alattar & Mendes de Leon, 2019).

Efforts to establish a comprehensive and effective MHPSS System in the KRI are met by a number of significant gaps and challenges. These include a shortage of qualified MHPSS professionals, insufficient capacity-building initiatives, a lack of MHPSS facilities and services, insufficient support from governmental bodies, or a lack of specialized services (Ahmed, 2022). This is all in light of the population's constantly increasing mental health needs. Another issue arises because most NGOs focus their psychosocial assistance efforts on IDP camps in the KRI. However, over 65% of displaced people reside outside of camps, as many have settled temporary housing in incomplete apartment complexes. This makes it difficult to identify and assist these groups, forcing them to rely on their own initiative to seek out psychiatric care from public clinics in major cities (EPIC, 2017). Moreover, it is crucial to acknowledge that MHPSS interventions may not always prevent the onset of PTSD or severe chronic mental illnesses. PM+, for example, is not appropriate for those who have severe mental health problems, such as those who are psychotic or suicidal (Dawson et al., 2015). In these cases, professional intervention by trained psychiatrists or psychotherapists is recommended, but this expertise is in short supply in Iraq (Kizilhan, 2021).

References

Abdallah, L. A. S., Abdel Aziz, T., Ali, N. I., Ali, S. H. T., Alkhoja, G. N., Bahnson, C., Dahdah, S., Dajani, I. K. Z., Denizer, A. C., Minatelli, J. L., Esen, F., Fotovat Ahmadi, S., Hart, T., Jaffrin, G. S., Jennings, R. S., Jokanovic, I., Kamphuis, B., Krishnan, N., Kulaksiz, S., . . . Onder, H. (2015). *The Kurdistan region of Iraq : assessing the economic and social impact of the Syrian conflict and ISIS (English)*. World Bank Group. http://documents.worldbank.org/curated/en/579451468305943474/The-Kurdistan-region-of-Iraq-assessing-the-economic-and-social-impact-of-the-Syrian-conflict-and-ISIS

Ahmed, D. R. (2022). Assessment of mental health and psychosocial support limitations, needs, and recommendations in Iraq. *Intervention, 20*(2), 193-194.

Akhtar, A., Giardinelli, L., Bawaneh, A., Awwad, M., Naser, H., Whitney, C., Jordans, M. J., Sijbrandij, M., Bryant, R. A., & Consortium, S.

(2020). Group problem management plus (gPM+) in the treatment of common mental disorders in Syrian refugees in a Jordanian camp: study protocol for a randomized controlled trial. *BMC Public Health*, *20*, 1-8.

Al Hilfi, T. K. (2014). Toward a healthier Iraq. *Yale Journal of Biology and Medicine*, *87*(3), 289-297.

Al Hilfi, T. K., Lafta, R., & Burnham, G. (2013). Health services in Iraq. *The Lancet*, *381*(9870), 939-948. https://doi.org/10.1016/S0140-6736(13)60320-7

Al Janabi, T., & Chung, S. (2022). Current Impact and Long-Term Influence of the COVID-19 Pandemic on Iraqi Healthcare Systems: A Case Study. *Epidemiologia*, *3*(4), 412-433. https://www.mdpi.com/2673-3986/3/4/32

Al Shawi, A. F., & Hassen, S. M. (2022). Traumatic events, post-traumatic stress disorders, and gender among Yazidi population after ISIS invasion: A post conflict study in Kurdistan – Iraq. *International Journal of Social Psychiatry*, *68*(3), 656-661. https://doi.org/10.1177/0020764021994145

Al-Bayan Center for Planning and Studies. (2018). *Restoring the Iraqi Healthcare Sector: The British National Health Service as a Model*. https://www.bayancenter.org/en/wp-content/uploads/2018/06/786564532.pdf

Al-Jumaili, A. A., Younus, M. M., Kannan, Y. J. A., Nooruldeen, Z. E., & Al-Nuseirat, A. (2021). Pharmaceutical regulations in Iraq: from medicine approval to postmarketing. *Eastern Mediterranean Health Journal*, *27*(10), 1007-1015. https://doi.org/10.26719/emhj.21.025

Al-Khalisi, N. (2013). The Iraqi medical brain drain: A cross-sectional study. *International Journal of Health Services*, *43*(2), 363-378. https://doi.org/10.2190/HS.43.2.j

Al-Salihy, Z., & Rahim, T. A. (2013). Mental health in the Kurdistan region of Iraq. *The Arab Journal of Psychiatry*, *44*(873), 1-4. https://doi.org/https://doi.org/10.12816/0001375

Alattar, Z., & Mendes de Leon, C. F. (2019). Task-Shifting Approaches to Refugee Mental Health in the Middle East: Literature Review. *ACCESS Health Journal*(4), 79-90. https://www.researchgate.net/profile/Juliann-Phd/publication/348480676_Final_ACCESS_Health_Journal_Spring_2019/links/60009a9845851553a0421258/Final-ACCESS-Health-Journal-Spring-2019.pdf#page=79

Ali, H., & Ari, K. (2021). Addressing Mental Health and Psychosocial Needs in Displacement: How a Stateless Person from Syria Became a

Refugee and Community Helper in Iraq [Personal Reflection]. *Intervention*, *19*(1), 136-140. https://doi.org/10.4103/intv.Intv_46_20

Alwan, A. (2004). *Health in Iraq: The current situation, our vision for the future and areas of work*. Ministry of Health.

Aziz, C. (2003). Struggling to rebuild Iraq's health-care system. War, sanctions, and mismanagement have left health system in shambles. *Lancet*, *362*(9392), 1288-1289. https://doi.org/10.1016/s0140-6736(03)14618-1

Beckmann, J., Wenzel, T., Hautzinger, M., & Kizilhan, J. I. (2022). Training of psychotherapists in post-conflict regions: A Community case study in the Kurdistan Region of Iraq [Community Case Study]. *Frontiers in Psychiatry*, *13*. https://doi.org/10.3389/fpsyt.2022.947903

Blackwell, M. A., Yeater, E. A., Ahmad, S., & Selmo, P. (2022). Sustaining psychotherapist effectiveness and independence: An exploratory study with displaced persons in Kurdistan, Iraq. *Traumatology*. https://doi.org/https://doi.org/10.1037/trm0000417

Böge, K., Hahn, E., Strasser, J., Schweininger, S., Bajbouj, M., & Karnouk, C. (2022). Psychotherapy in the Kurdistan region of Iraq (KRI): Preferences and expectations of the Kurdish host community, internally displaced- and Syrian refugee community. *International Journal of Social Psychiatry*, *68*(2), 346-353. https://doi.org/10.1177/0020764021995219

Bolton, P. (2013). Mental health in Iraq: issues and challenges. *Lancet*, *381*(9870), 879-881. https://doi.org/10.1016/s0140-6736(13)60637-6

Bolton, P. (2019). 1 - Global mental health and psychotherapy: Importance of task-shifting and a systematic approach to adaptation. In D. J. Stein, J. K. Bass, & S. G. Hofmann (Eds.), *Global Mental Health and Psychotherapy* (pp. 11-24). Academic Press. https://doi.org/https://doi.org/10.1016/B978-0-12-814932-4.00001-X

Bradley, M. (2016). *Iraq's Doctors Face Threats of Violence*. The Wall Street Journal. Retrieved 01.08.23 from https://www.wsj.com/articles/iraqs-doctors-face-threats-of-violence-1462145946

Cetorelli, V., & Shabila, N. P. (2014). Expansion of health facilities in Iraq a decade after the US-led invasion, 2003–2012. *Conflict and Health*, *8*(1), 16. https://doi.org/10.1186/1752-1505-8-16

Collins, P. Y., Patel, V., Joestl, S. S., March, D., Insel, T. R., Daar, A. S., Anderson, W., Dhansay, M. A., Phillips, A., Shurin, S., Walport, M., Ewart, W., Savill, S. J., Bordin, I. A., Costello, E. J., Durkin, M., Fairburn, C., Glass, R. I., Hall, W., . . . Stein, D. J. (2011). Grand challenges in global mental health. *Nature*, *475*(7354), 27-30. https://doi.org/10.1038/475027a

Dawson, K. S., Bryant, R. A., Harper, M., Tay, A. K., Rahman, A., Schafer, A., & Van Ommeren, M. (2015). Problem Management Plus (PM+): a WHO transdiagnostic psychological intervention for common mental health problems. *World Psychiatry*, *14*(3), 354.

Duran, D., & Menon, R. (2020). *Mitigating the Impact of COVID-19 and Strengthening Health Systems in the Middle East and North Africa*. World Bank. http://hdl.handle.net/10986/34238

EPIC. (2017). *Iraq's Quiet Mental Health Crisis*. Enabling Peace in Iraq Center. Retrieved 08.08.23 from https://www.epic-usa.org/iraq-mental-health/

Finnish Immigration Service. (2019). *Iraq: Fact-Finding Mission to Baghdad in February 2019; Mental Health Issues and Their Treatment in Iraq*. https://www.ecoi.net/en/file/local/2037739/Iraq-FFM-report-Mental-Health-Issues.pdf

Godichet, O., & Ghanem, V. (2004). Iraqi system of primary health care: a communitarian system of family medicine under a dictatorship framework. *Contemporary Nurse*, *17*(1-2), 113-124. https://doi.org/10.5172/conu.17.1-2.113

Halaj, A., & Huppert, J. D. (2017). Middle East. In S. G. Hofmann (Ed.), *International Perspectives on Psychotherapy* (pp. 219-239). Springer International Publishing. https://doi.org/10.1007/978-3-319-56194-3_11

Henderson, A. E., & United States Institute of, P. (2005). *The Coalition Provisional Authority's experience with economic reconstruction in Iraq: lessons learned*. United States Institute of Peace. http://hdl.handle.net/2027/pur1.32754077956724

Humphreys, K., & Sadik, S. (2006). Rebuilding Iraq's mental health system. *Behavioral Healthcare*, *26*(7), 34-35.

Husni, M., Taylor, F., & Koye, N. (2006). Medical education and health care in Iraqi Kurdistan in the last four decades. *Medicine, Conflict and Survival*, *22*(4), 292-298. https://doi.org/10.1080/13623690600945214

IOM Iraq. (2023). *Mental Health and Psychosocial Support Programme: Activities Overview (January – December 2022)*. https://reliefweb.int/attachments/d1eec035-1cbb-4492-a019-47108becc019/iom_iraq_mhpss_activitiesoverview_januarydecember2022_digital.pdf

IRFAD. (2014). *Healthcare in Iraq*. Retrieved 01.08.23 from www.irfad.org/healthcare-in-iraq

Kapp, C. (2003). Anarchy pushes Iraqi health system to brink of collapse. *Lancet*, *361*(9366), 1351. https://doi.org/10.1016/s0140-6736(03)13089-9

Karadaghi, G., & Willott, C. (2015). Doctors as the governing body of the Kurdish health system: exploring upward and downward accountability among physicians and its influence on the adoption of coping behaviours. *Human Resources for Health*, *13*(1), 43. https://doi.org/10.1186/s12960-015-0039-x

Kizilhan, J. I. (2020). Stress on local and international psychotherapists in the crisis region of Iraq. *BMC Psychiatry*, *20*, 1-8.

Kizilhan, J. I. (2021). Mental Health in Crisis Regions. In J. A. Chambers (Ed.), *Field Guide to Global Health & Disaster Medicine*. Elsevier Health Sciences.

Kizilhan, J. I., Friedl, N., Neumann, J., & Traub, L. (2020). Potential trauma events and the psychological consequences for Yazidi women after ISIS captivity. *BMC Psychiatry*, *20*(1), 256. https://doi.org/10.1186/s12888-020-02671-4

Kok, D. J., Maghdid, D. M., Mohammed, M. S., & Sherwani, G. H. (2014). Academic development for urologists in the Kurdistan region of Iraq. *Arab Journal of Urology*, *12*(1), 79-82. https://doi.org/10.1016/j.aju.2013.08.003

Koya University. (2017). *Koya University facilitates a mental health and psychological support center*. Retrieved 01.08.23 from http://koyauniversity.org/ar/node/138

Kurdistan Board of Medical Specialities. (2018). *About Us*. Kurdistan Board of Medical Specialities. Retrieved 01.08.23 from https://khcms.edu.krd/?page=aboutus

Kurdistan Regional Government. (2021). *List of licensed projects in Kurdistan region*. https://govkrd.b-cdn.net/OtherEntities/Board%20of%20Investment/English/Publication/Licensed%20Projects/List%20of%20Licensed%20Projects%20in%20Kurdistan%20Region.pdf

Kurdistan Regional Government. (2023a). *Kurdistan Region a shelter for about one million refugees and IDPs*. Kurdistan Regional Government,. Retrieved 09.08.23 from https://gov.krd/dmi-en/activities/news-and-press-releases/2023/january/kurdistan-region-a-shelter-for-about-one-million-refugees-and-idps/

Kurdistan Regional Government. (2023b). *Kurdistan Region is a great environment for NGO activities*. Kurdistan Regional Government, . Retrieved 03.08.23 from https://gov.krd/dmi-en/activities/news-and-press-releases/2023/february/kurdistan-region-is-a-great-environment-for-ngo-activities/

Kurdistan Regional Government. (2024). *Kurdistan Fact Sheet*. Kurdistan Regional Government,. Retrieved 09.08.24 from https://gov.krd/boi-en/why-kurdistan/region/facts-figures/region-kurdistan-fact-sheet/

Mahmood, H. N., Ibrahim, H., Ismail, A. A., & Neuner, F. (2022). Does Time Heal Trauma? 18 Month Follow-Up Study of Syrian Refugees'

Mental Health in Iraq's Kurdistan Region. *International Journal of Environmental Research and Public Health*, *19*(22). https://doi.org/10.3390/ijerph192214910

Middle East Research Institute. (2015). *Health System Challenges in the Face of the Humanitarian Crisis in Iraq*. MERI. Retrieved 01.08.23 from http://www.meri-k.org/health-system-challenges-in-the-face-of-the-humanitarian-crisis-in-iraq-full/

Ministry of Interior Joint Crisis Coordination Center. *Common Operational Picture: Humanitarian Respone in the Kurdistan Region of Iraq*. https://jcckrg.org/contents/reports/25-10-2016/1477385146.COP%20-%20Issue%20No%206-%20January%202016.pdf

Ministry of Planning. (2010). *National Development Plan for the years 2010–14*. https://planipolis.iiep.unesco.org/sites/default/files/ressources/iraq_national_development_plan_2010-2014.pdf

Mukdarut, B., Lambert, F., & Kelly, D. (2019). Mental health and psychosocial support programmes for adults in humanitarian emergencies: a systematic review and meta-analysis in low and middle-income countries. *BMJ Global Health*, *4*(5), e001484. https://doi.org/10.1136/bmjgh-2019-001484

Murakami, N. J., & Akilova, M. (2022). *Integrative Social Work Practice with Refugees, Asylum Seekers, and Other Forcibly Displaced Persons*. Cham Springer International Publishing AG 2022. http://lib.ugent.be/catalog/ebk01:2548350800004l

Musotsi, P., Koyiet, P., Khoshaba, N., Ali, A., Elias, F., Abdulmaleek, M., Simiyu, K., & Rosenkranz, E. (2022). Highlighting Complementary Benefits of Problem Management Plus (PM+) and Doing What Matters in Times of Stress (DWM) Interventions Delivered Alongside Broader Community MHPSS Programming in Zummar, Ninewa Governorate of Iraq [Article]. *Intervention*, *20*(2), 139-150. https://doi.org/10.4103/intv.intv_7_22

Price, R. A. (2018). *Iraqi State Capabilities*. https://core.ac.uk/download/pdf/286048575.pdf

Pring, C. (2015). *Kurdistan Region of Iraq: Overview of corruption and anti-corruption*. http://www.transparency.org/files/content/corruptionqas/Kurdistan_Region_of_Iraq_overview_of_corruption_and_anti-corruption_2015.pdf

Sadik, S., & Al-Jadiry, A. M. (2006). Mental health services in Iraq: past, present and future. *Psychiatry International*, *3*(4), 11-13.

Saleh, A. M., Shabila, N. P., Dabbagh, A. A., Al-Tawil, N. G., & Al-Hadithi, T. S. (2015). A qualitative assessment of faculty perspectives of small group teaching experience in Iraq. *BMC Medical Education*, *15*(1), 19. https://doi.org/10.1186/s12909-015-0304-7

Shabila, N. P., Al-Tawil, N. G., Tahir, R., Shwani, F. H., Saleh, A. M., & Al-Hadithi, T. S. (2010). Iraqi health system in kurdistan region: medical professionals' perspectives on challenges and priorities for improvement. *Conflict and Health*, *4*, 19. https://doi.org/10.1186/1752-1505-4-19

Shukor, A. R., Klazinga, N. S., & Kringos, D. S. (2017). Primary care in an unstable security, humanitarian, economic and political context: the Kurdistan Region of Iraq. *BMC Health Services Research*, *17*(1), 592. https://doi.org/10.1186/s12913-017-2501-z

Syrian Civic Platform. (2018). *Syrian Refugees in the Kurdistan Region of Iraq: Harsh Conditions and Marginalization*. https://www.scplatform.net/en/wp-content/uploads/2018/11/Syrian-Refugees-in-the-Kurdistan-Region-of-Iraq-.pdf

Taha, P. H., & Sijbrandij, M. (2021). Gender Differences in Traumatic Experiences, PTSD, and Relevant Symptoms among the Iraqi Internally Displaced Persons. *International Journal of Environmental Research and Public Health*, *18*(18). https://doi.org/10.3390/ijerph18189779

Tawfik-Shukor, A., & Khoshnaw, H. (2010). The impact of health system governance and policy processes on health services in Iraqi Kurdistan. *BMC International Health and Human Rights*, *10*(1), 14. https://doi.org/10.1186/1472-698X-10-14

UN Habitat. (2024). *Iraq Risk Reduction and Rehabilitation*. UN Habitat. Retrieved 10.08.24 from https://unhabitat.org/iraq-risk-reduction-and-rehabilitation

UNHCR. (2022). *Iraq Factsheet, September 2022*. https://reporting.unhcr.org/iraq-factsheet-3461

UNHCR. (2023a). *3RP Iraq Country Chapter 2023-2024*. https://data2.unhcr.org/en/documents/details/101217

UNHCR. (2023b). *Irap 2022 - Populations*. UNHCR. Retrieved 09.08.23 from https://reporting.unhcr.org/operational/operations/iraq?page=0&year=2022#toc-populations

United Nations. (2022). *Syrian refugees in Iraq, risk losing access to basic food supplies*. UN News. Retrieved 09.08.23 from https://news.un.org/en/story/2022/05/1118472

United Nations High Commissioner for Refugees. (2014). *3RP Regional Refugee and Resilience Plan 2015–2016 in Response to the Syria Crisis*. https://reliefweb.int/attachments/1858eae4-5e1c-3b96-a7b1-c6df1a9572a6/3RP2015AnnualReport.pdf

United Nations Iraq. (2022). *Iraq Common Country Analysis (2022—Condensed Version).* https://iraq.un.org/sites/default/files/2022-07/CCA%20Iraq%20-%20Condensed.pdf

United Nations Office of the Iraq Programme Oil-for-Food. (2004a). *Implementation of the Oil for Food: a chronology*. Retrieved 01.08.23 from http://www.un.org/Depts/oip/background/chron.html

United Nations Office of the Iraq Programme Oil-for-Food. (2004b). *Roles and Responsibilities of United Nations Bodies at Work in Northern Iraq*. Retrieved 01.08.23 from http://www.un.org/Depts/oip/north.html

UNOCHA. (2018). *Humanitarian Needs Overview 2019 – Iraq*. https://www.humanitarianresponse.info/sites/www.humanitarianresponse.info/files/documents/files/2019_hno_irq_28122018.pdf

Womersley, G., & Arikut-Treece, Y. (2019). Collective trauma among displaced populations in Northern Iraq: A case study evaluating the therapeutic interventions of the Free Yezidi Foundation [Article]. *Intervention*, *17*(1), 3-12. https://doi.org/10.4103/intv.Intv_56_18

World Bank. *Data for Iraq: Hospital beds (per 1,000 people)*. Retrieved 01.08.23 from https://data.worldbank.org/indicator/SH.MED.BEDS.ZS?locations=IQ

World Health Organization. (2006). *Iraq Health System Profile*. https://www.ecoi.net/en/file/local/1234809/1228_1216905471_irak.pdf

World Health Organization. (2016a). *MHPSS Situation Analysis: Anbar province and KRG, Iraq*. https://www.google.com/url?sa=t&rct=j&q=&esrc=s&source=web&cd=&cad=rja&uact=8&ved=2ahUKEwjT-4KSrcCAAxXM6aQKHQ3OAvgQFnoECA8QAQ&url=https%3A%2F%2Fwww.mhinnovation.net%2Fsites%2Fdefault%2Ffiles%2Fdownloads%2Fresource%2FWHO.UNHCR%2520KRG.Iraq%25202015%2520MHPSS%2520Situation%2520Analysis%2520KRG.docx&usg=AOvVaw06QjAmmNUY4mmacnMNhK8c&opi=89978449

World Health Organization. (2016b). *Problem management plus (PM+): individual psychological help for adults impaired by distress in communities exposed to adversity* (7521738403).

World Health Organization. (2020). *Mental health atlas country profile: Iraq*. https://cdn.who.int/media/docs/default-source/mental-health/mental-health-atlas-2020-country-profiles/irq.pdf?sfvrsn=641f2b5e_7&download=true

World Health Organization. (2023). *The Global Health Observatory*. Retrieved 01.08.23 from https://www.who.int/data/gho

World Health Organization. (2024). *Health System Strengthening*. Retrieved 23.08.24 from https://www.emro.who.int/iraq/priority-areas/health-system-strengthening.html

World Health Organization. Regional Office for the Eastern, M. (2022). *World Health Organization Iraq annual report 2021*. World Health Organization. Regional Office for the Eastern Mediterranean. https://apps.who.int/iris/handle/10665/361313

Wörmer, N., & Lamberty, L. (2018). *Scattered Dreams: The Independence Referendum, the Fall of Kirkuk and the Effect on Kurdish and Iraqi Politics*. K. A. Stiftung. https://www.kas.de/documents/252038/253252/7_dokument_dok_pdf_52122_2.pdf/0a606c42-1abd-1641-9b4d-44d6cd25eca8?version=1.0&t=1539647624437

Younis, M. S., & Khunda, D. (2020). A personal history of psychiatry in Iraq through war and conflict. *Global Psychiatry*. https://doi.org/10.2478/gp-2020-0017

Zarocostas, J. (2007). Exodus of medical staff strains Iraq's health facilities. *Bmj*, *334*(7599), 865. https://doi.org/10.1136/bmj.39195.466713.DB

CHAPTER 6

YAZIDI HISTORY, SOCIETY, RELIGION AND TRAUMA

JAN ILHAN KIZILHAN

The next chapter explores the Yazidi religion, along with the social structure of the community and its history. This chapter is also part of the context and needs assessment that preceded the foundation of the Institute for Psychotherapy and Psychotraumatology (IPP). Identifying vulnerable groups and understanding their needs is crucial for the successful implementation of healthcare projects such as the Duhok project.

Short Introduction to Yazidism

The word "Yazidi", or variations "Yezidi", "Izîdî" or "Ezdayi", "Êzîdî", as it is pronounced by the members of the religious community, comes from the Kurdish language and means "the one who created me", referring to the Creator and God (Kreyenbroek & Jindī, 2005). Throughout this text, I will use the term "Yazidi" for consistency, as it has been used for several centuries and is the most widely recognized by the general public.

Yazidism embodies the belief in a singular Entity and in one God, representing a monotheistic faith (Omarkhali, 2017). The Yazidi call God "Xweda" (Khuda), which means "the one who created himself" (Grant, 1915). Aligned with theological tenets shared by Judaism, Christianity, and Islam, Yazidi daily prayers encompass the veneration of seven archangels. The chief of the seven angels is Tausi Melek, the Peacock Angel. Tausi Melek is entrusted by God with overseeing the world and specifically protecting the Yazidi people (Hunter, 2017). Each Yazidi is obliged to an annual three-day fast in December, as a sign of gratitude for the creation of the earth and in remembrance of God and the Yazidi faith. Additionally, each Yazidi must visit the holy temple "Lalish" in northern Iraq at least once in their lifetime. The Yazidi faith includes a system of beliefs with universal principles on ethics and morals, right and wrong, justice, truth, loyalty, mercy, and love (Guest, 2012).

The History of the Yazidi

The Yazidi consider themselves to be members of one of the world's oldest religions and often make reference to Mithraism and its relationship to Yarsan and Zarathrustra (Kreyenbroek & Jindī, 2005). The Yazidi have reported experiencing massacres since the Arab invasion of the Near and Middle East in 637 A.D., which led to enforced Islamization. These atrocities have persisted into the present day. Yazidi people were, and continue to be, labeled by radical Muslims as "Devil Worshippers" and are not recognized as "Followers of the Book." Confronted with the pressure to embrace Islam, Yazidi people sought refuge in the hills, limiting their interactions with other groups.

Their religion has been passed down orally by priests, making the history of the Yazidi an "Oral History" (Kizilhan, 2014). There are very few written documents about the Yazidi, and this has only begun to change in the last 50 years (Furlani, 1936; Omarkhali, 2017). The Yazidi generally assume that their origins trace back to the Mithraic religion, up to the 14th century B.C. However, there is no mention of the term 'Yazidi' in historical sources until the 7th century A.D. Around the turn of the century, Muslim clerics and historians started using the term "Yazidi" (Al-Damalgi, 1949).

In the 10th century, the Arabian historian Al-Samani (ca. 1166) described the Yazidi as a group of Aztecs living in the Helwan hills (now known as northern Iraq/the Kurdistan Region), in his book "Al-Ansab" (The Genealogies). In his book he also mentions that the Yazidi are loyal to Yazid Ibn Muawiya, the second Ommayid Caliph (Al-Samani, 1912). In some communities in Kurdish regions, this false belief is still held today and has often been used as a justification for plundering and enslaving the Yazidi. Since that time, and even today, some Shiites and Alevites believe that the Yazidi, as followers of Yazid Ibn Muawiya, killed the prophet Ali's sons Hasan and Hüssein, who were intended to be Mohammed's successors. It is only in the last forty years that there has been any real contact between the Yazidi and the Alevites, and they are engaged in dialogue today (Iranica, 2014). When the Ottoman Empire collapsed, many Yazidis, along with the Armenians, fled to present-day Armenia and settled in the Caucasus regions of the former Soviet Union. At the end of the First World War and the foundation of Turkey in 1923, the Yazidi homeland was partitioned. Since then, the Yazidi have been living in Turkey, Iraq, Syria, and the former Soviet Union.

Sheikh Adi and the Founding of a New System of Religion

In recent years the last Yazidi reformer, Sheikh Adi, has repeatedly been the subject of discussions within the Yazidi community. Given the Yazidi are forbidden from having relationships and marrying people of different religions, they are very critical of Islam. In the past, the Yazidi have suffered countless reprisals and persecution, and have had to flee from Muslims on many occasions. It is claimed that Sheikh Adi himself was a Muslim, but many Yazidi reject this claim, asserting that one can only be Yazidi by birth. The religious and ethnic origin of Sheikh Adi is still the subject of numerous discussions in the Yezidi community. The religious leaders of the Yezidis avoid talking about this topic because, from their religious point of view, no Muslim is allowed to become a Yezidi and lead them. Unlike Christianity or Islam, there were no Yazidi missionaries to recruit others.

Countless documents confirm that Sheikh Adi, son of Musafir, was born in the village of Bait al-Far (known as Khirbet Qanfar today), in the Baalbak region of Lebanon, around 1050 or 1075. He is a descendant of the Ibrahim family, son of Abdul Malik and Mervan IbnAl-Hakam (Al-Jazri, 1966). Sheikh Adi died aged ninety. The Yazidi regard Sheikh Adi as the incarnation of Tausi Melek, the Peacock Angel. The Tal Lalish became Sheikh Adi's headquarters and since that time has been regarded as holy, becoming a place of pilgrimage for all Yazidi (Kreyenbroek & Jindī, 2005). At that time, the Yazidi believed that Sheikh Adi received his mental and spiritual power from Tausi Melek (the Peacock Angel). The oral tradition also says that Sheikh Adi was sent by Tausi Melek to be the leader of the Yazidi (Kreyenbroek & Jindī, 2005). After settling among the Yazidi, he introduced a new religious doctrine called "Sad u Had", which translates to "Rights and Duties" (Kizilhan, 1997).

The Caste System

Sheikh Adi's arrival amongst the Yazidi community in the 12th century had significance beyond religious aspects. Setting up the caste system changed the whole structure of the community and relationships between the groups were redefined. There were the *Sheikhs* (teachers) on the one hand, and the *Murids* (lay people, the people) on the other. This structure is also observed among the Sufis. The existing group of priests (*Pirs*) lost their position as the main instructors in the Yazidi religion. However, they were so strongly anchored in the Yazidi community that they continued to play an important religious role, albeit subordinate to the Sheikhs (Kizilhan, 2009; Lescot, 1938).

The Yazidi tribes were divided between the Sheikhs and Pirs. Each Sheikh and Pir who was responsible for a tribe had to have a connection to the instructor of the other tribes (Kreyenbroek & Jindī, 2005). Marriage between Pir and Sheikh castes is forbidden. Within the Sheikh caste, individuals are only allowed to marry descendants from their own group. In the Pir caste, it is a taboo for persons descending from Pir Hasan to marry Mamans. The Pirs can, however, marry among their own people. It is strictly forbidden for Murids to marry Sheikhs or Pirs (Jindy, 1998; Omarkhali, 2017).

The marriage prohibitions between castes create clear social boundaries (Al-Jadan, 1960). It is only possible to be a member of a group by birth and it is not possible to change groups. Such a clear division, and the fact that it is impossible to change to a different caste, prevents any power struggle between the castes. Each individual is aware of their social status and has no opportunity to change this. Marrying a person from a different religious community is also not possible.

Many of these rules have been destroyed as a result of the terror carried out by ISIS in 2014, including the rape of thousands of women, young girls, and children. Sexual contact with non-Yazidi individuals led to the community rejecting its own daughters and wives, since they were no longer considered Yazidi. In addition to destroying physical infrastructure, the ISIS terrorist group is systematically trying to destroy a whole community, which is why the UN refers to this as genocide (United Nations, 2017).

Collective Trauma and Terror

The Islamization of the Kurdish areas in Iraq, Iran, Syria, and Turkey led to a long history of persecution. The Kurds, including the Yazidi, were forced to convert to Islam. This did not occur with the onset of ISIS terror, but with the overall Islamization of the Middle East. It is estimated that 74 genocides have been carried out against the Yazidi in the past 800 years by Islamized groups and states. To date, according to conservative estimates, approximately 1.8 million Yazidi have had to convert to Islam and approximately 1.2 million Yazidi have been killed (Gerdau et al., 2017; Kizilhan, 2017b). Numerous fatwas have "legitimized" their killing, looting, abduction, and forcible conversion to Islam. ISIS uses that as a spurious argument to carry out genocide against the Yazidi (Kizilhan & Othman, 2012).

Minority religions such as Yazidi, oriental Christians, Mandaeans, Shabaks, Feylis, and other groups have often been the target of persecution and annihilation by radical Islamized groups in the Middle East (Gerdau et al., 2017). After the end of the Saddam Hussein era in 2003, and particularly since 2007, hundreds of Yazidi people have been murdered by the terrorist group Al-Qaida in Iraq (Kizilhan & Othman, 2012). Even today they are ostracized and have to suffer reprisals from the Muslim majority. Since the attack by ISIS at the beginning of August 2014, more than 7,000 Yazidi have been killed, thousands of families have been held hostage in their villages and, if they did not convert to Islam, they were murdered. Over 5,800 young girls have been abducted, raped, sold on Arab markets, enslaved or killed. Over 20,000 Yazidi have fled to Syria, 30,000 to Turkey, and over 360,000 to the Kurdish region. The Yazidi have been, and are still being, systematically persecuted and murdered (Tekin et al., 2016).

Systematic Destruction of the Yazidi Community

From the 3rd of August 2014 onwards, ISIS began terrorizing Yazidi villages and soon gained control of the area. The Iraqi army and the Kurdish Peshmerga retreated and the people were helpless, at the mercy of ISIS terror. People were herded into buildings such as schools and town halls, and their jewelry and valuables were stolen. IS then separated the men from the women and many men were executed immediately. More than 150 women who I interviewed reported that in the village of Kocho, for example, over 413 men were executed on the 15th of August in 2014 After that, older women, women with children, married women without children, and young boys and girls between eight and 14 years old, were grouped together and taken to various locations. Older women and women with children were interned in mass accommodation or villages, near Tel-Afar or Mosul, where the Shiites had previously lived. They were guarded by IS fighters, humiliated, beaten, and raped. Every evening, male civilians from Syria, Saudi Arabia, Egypt, Qatar, Tunisia, and other countries arrived because they wanted to buy the women and take them away (Cetorelli et al., 2017).

Women are being forced to convert to Islam and to pray in Arabic every day, even though they only speak Kurdish. Children are being drilled and exploited, like African child-soldiers. They are being brought up to be brutal, even towards their own families. In camps, children are trained to beat other children, crucify them, or bury them alive if they do not adhere to IS demands. Those who are not sent to fight serve as the emirs' lackeys, guards, or as spies in the villages or camps where Yazidi and other religious minorities are held captive (Kizilhan, 2017a).

Since the Yazidi do not see any hope of a peaceful life in Iraq, they are trying to leave the country. Many want to come to Germany because the Yazidi have been migrating from Turkey to Germany since the 1960s.

Flight and Migration

For more than 70 years, the Yazidi have been living in Germany as migrants who have left their homeland for economic and political reasons. According to some estimates, of the approximately 40,000 Yazidi who used to reside in Turkey, around 38,000 live in Germany today (Kizilhan, 2014). According to the Turkish interior ministry, there are now no more than 1570 Yazidi living in the whole of Turkey. Because of their small population number, the Yazidi can no longer live effectively as a group in Turkey or revitalize their community. Most of the 1570 Yazidi are over 60 years old, and the majority of the next generation live in Europe.

In recent years, increasing numbers of Yazidi have also fled to Germany from Syria, Iraq, and the former Soviet Union. Since the IS invasion in 2014, approximately 40,000 Yazidi have fled to Germany from Iraq alone. There are approximately 150,000 Yazidi in Germany and a further 60,000 in the other European countries, with population numbers continuing to increase (Kizilhan, 2017b). Around 20,000 Yazidi are now living in the USA, 8,000 in Canada, and 6,000 in Australia. Since Europe is completely foreign to the Yazidi, they are exposed to many social, political, and cultural difficulties. The way of life is different for the new, severely traumatized Yazidi.

Yazidi refugee children and adolescents do not just suffer from PTSD, but from various other problems as well (Tekin et al., 2016). As such, issues faced by survivors of torture need to be understood more broadly, beyond just PTSD symptoms. It is important to consider the broader context of their experience, including their status as asylum seekers or refugees, their ethnic background, and various psychological and social health factors (Kizilhan, 2017b). In addition to mental disorders like PTSD, long-term studies indicate that there have been changes in the social, cultural, and religious structures of the community following migration due to the IS. The Yazidi community has been fundamentally changed and it is not clear whether they will survive as group. They can learn from the trauma they have experienced and can grow as a group by adapting new rules in the wake of migration. This includes revisiting rules relating to marriage to non-Yazidis, changing the caste system, and trying to overcome collective and individual trauma.

Conclusions

The extent to which trauma management is feasible also depends on the way a society deals with the topics of sexuality, violence, and transgenerational stress. Women have been raped and abused, and this is publicly known. In this context, the women experience considerable insecurity and sometimes refuse to talk about their experiences as it is a complete taboo topic. High moral conceptions and limitations, along with internalized attitudes relating to "honor and the violation of honor," lead to considerable worry and the fear of collective exclusion among these women. In this respect, feelings of shame play a particular role. This is because, in a "shame culture," the focus is not primarily on the incident itself or the actual violation of norms. Instead, the emphasis is on how one can preserve their reputation in front of others. For example, the rape of a young woman can be considered as disgraceful by the collective and the victim can be ostracized, clearly demonstrating issues faced beyond the traumatic event itself.

The catastrophe of 2014 has led to a break in society. The loss suffered and the unclear future are being compensated for by looking for a new identity than the previous one in order to survive. These changes take a long time to take effect. On the other hand, some individuals who are freed from their old rites and rules may have difficulties in feeling at ease in their new "religious homeland". This new homeland, however, can provide a real chance of survival for the following generation. Renewals, reforms, and changes do not necessarily need to be negative or problematical experiences. It is possible that the growing cosmopolitan nature of society, along with migration and exposure to other cultures, can be seen as enriching experiences and may therefore facilitate processes of renewal for the Yazidi. Reorientation and transformation are necessary, but are only possible once the historical and individual trauma has been processed.

References

Al-Damalgi, S. (1949). The Yazidi. *Al-Itihad Press, Mousil.*

Al-Jadan, K. (1960). *Cate among the Yazidi* MA Thesis in Rural Sociology. The Pennsylvania State University Press].

Al-Jazri, A. (1966). The Complete in History. *Beirut: Sader Press.[Paper reference 1].*

Al-Samani, A. (1912). *Al Ansab (Arabic: The Lineage)*. Brill, E.J. Press.

Cetorelli, V., Sasson, I., Shabila, N., & Burnham, G. (2017). Mortality and kidnapping estimates for the Yazidi population in the area of Mount Sinjar, Iraq, in August 2014: A retrospective household survey. *PLoS medicine*, *14*(5), e1002297.

Furlani, G. (1936). I santi dei Yezidi. *Orientalia*, *5*, 64-83.

Gerdau, I., Kizilhan, J. I., & Noll-Hussong, M. (2017). Posttraumatic stress disorder and related disorders among female Yazidi refugees following Islamic state of Iraq and Syria attacks—a case series and mini-review. *Frontiers in Psychiatry*, *8*, 282.

Grant, A. (1915). *The Nestrians or the Lost Tribes*. Philadelphia Press.

Guest, J. S. (2012). *Survival among the Kurds*. Routledge.

Hunter, E. C. (2017). Religious minorities of the modern middle east: a complete survey of non-muslim communities.

Iranica, E. (2014). *Yazidis*. Retrieved 26.04.2024 from https://www.iranicaonline.org/articles/yazidis-i-general-

Jindy, K. (1998). Naḥwa Ma ʻrifat Ḥaqīqat al-Diyānat al-Īzīdiyya. In: Towards a Knowledge of the Truth of Yezidi Religion], Uppsala.

Kizilhan, I. (1997). *Die Yeziden: eine anthropologische und sozialpsychologische Studie über die kurdische Gemeinschaft*. Verlag Medico International. https://books.google.de/books?id=Hnq6AAAAIAAJ

Kizilhan, J., & Othman, M. (2012). Trauma nach einer Bombenexplosion im Irak PTSD-Faktoren bei Opfern der gropten Bombenexplosion im Irak im Jahre 2007.[Trauma after a Bomb Explosion in Iraq. PTSD Factors of the Survivors of the Bomb Explosion in 2007.]. *Zeitschrift Trauma & Gewalt*, *6*, 62-71.

Kizilhan, J. I. (2009). Die Yeziden. Between Tradition and Globalism. [The Yazidi. Between Tradition and Globalism.]. *Journal for Kurdish Studies. Kurdish Institut Paris.*

Kizilhan, J. I. (2014). *Verortete Erinnerungen in der Gegenwart: das religiöse und kulturelle Gedächtnis der Yeziden in der Türkei*. VWB, Verlag für Wissenschaft und Bildung.

Kizilhan, J. I. (2017a). Behandlung traumatisierter Frauen in Deutschland. *Forensische Psychiatrie Psychologie Kriminologie*, *11*(4), 335-341.

Kizilhan, J. I. (2017b). Treatment of traumatized women in Germany: Transcultural aspects exemplified by 1000 Yazidis from northern Iraq. *Forensische Psychiatrie, Psychologie, Kriminologie*, *11*, 335-341.

Kreyenbroek, P. G., & Jindī, K. (2005). *God and Sheikh Adi are perfect: sacred poems and religious narratives from the Yezidi tradition* (Vol. 9). Otto Harrassowitz Verlag.

Lescot, R. (1938). Enquête sur les Yezidis de Syrie et du Djebel Sindjār. *Mémoires de l'Institut Français de Damas*.

Omarkhali, K. (2017). *The Yezidi religious textual tradition: from oral to written: categories, transmission, scripturalisation and canonisation of the Yezidi oral religious texts: with samples of oral and written religious texts and with audio and video samples on CD-ROM*. Harrassowitz.

Tekin, A., Karadağ, H., Süleymanoğlu, M., Tekin, M., Kayran, Y., Alpak, G., & Şar, V. (2016). Prevalence and gender differences in symptomatology of posttraumatic stress disorder and depression among Iraqi Yazidis displaced into Turkey. *European journal of psychotraumatology*, *7*(1), 28556.

United Nations. (2017). *ISIL's 'genocide' against Yazidis is ongoing, UN rights panel says, calling for international action*. UN News. Retrieved 03.06.24 from https://news.un.org/en/story/2017/08/562772-isils-genocide-against-yazidis-ongoing-un-rights-panel-says-calling

PART 2

THE DUHOK PROJECT

CHAPTER 7

DESCRIPTION OF THE PILOT PROJECT

JAN ILHAN KIZILHAN, JULIA BECKMANN AND ANNA WEIGELT

This chapter will provide a comprehensive overview of "The Duhok Project," detailing the origins of the Institute for Psychotherapy and Psychotraumatology, its structural organization, and the curriculum and content of the Master of Advanced Studies in Psychotherapy and Psychotraumatology (MASPP) offered there. Additionally, the chapter will explore the institute's networking activities, research endeavors, initiatives founded by the IPP, and the challenges faced in the process of transferring responsibilities to ensure the institute's independence from international actors.

Origins of the Project

The idea for this project stemmed from two primary factors. Firstly, it was a response to the pressing health challenges prevailing in northern Iraq, as described in the preceding chapters of this book. Secondly, the initiative found its roots in the extensive history of conflict and suffering that has characterized the Kurdistan Region of Iraq (KRI) in general.

Kurdistan is a region in the Middle East that is home to the Kurdish people. After World War I and the fall of the Ottoman Empire, the Treaty of Sevres (1920) proposed an autonomous Kurdish state. However this proposal was rejected by the Turkish leader, Mustafa Kemal Ataturk. The Treaty of Lausanne (1923) later replaced the Treaty of Sevres, dividing Kurdistan among Turkey, Syria, Iran, and Iraq, leaving the Kurds as minorities in each of these countries. In the decades that followed, the Kurdish people faced repeated discrimination, persecution, armed conflicts, rebellions, and genocides in all four countries. Iraqi Kurdistan finally gained de facto autonomy from Iraq in 1991. In 2005, the Baghdad government officially recognized the autonomy of the region in its constitution.

The discrimination and persecution of the Kurds intensified in Iraq after the Ba'ath Party came into power in 1968. In an effort to "Arabize" the country from 1975 onwards, hundreds of Kurdish villages were destroyed, and thousands of people forcibly relocated (Black, 1993). During the Iran-Iraq War (1980-1988), Kurdish partisans (peshmerga) fought alongside Iran against the Iraqi forces. The Iraqi government, under Saddam Hussein, retaliated by launching the "Anfal" campaign in 1988 (Shorsh, 2007). The campaign included eight military offensives which targeted Kurdish people in northern Iraq from February 23rd to September 6th in 1988. The eight offensives included aerial bombing, systematic destruction of settlements, mass deportation, imprisonment, torture, firing squads, and chemical warfare. It is estimated that during the Anfal campaign, about 200,000 Kurdish people disappeared. More than 4,000 villages were destroyed including public places such as schools, mosques, and churches. Of the seven million livestock present in Kurdistan at the beginning of the Anfal campaign, only 50,000 remained after this attack (Bolton et al., 2013).

On March 16th, 1988, during the first Anfal offensive, the city of Halabja was subjected to a chemical attack involving multiple poisonous gases. This attack killed roughly 5,000 people in one day and left 10,000 injured (Karim & Baser, 2022). The victims were mostly civilians and, with their homes destroyed, most of those who fled never returned. The consequences of the attack, which are still noticeable today, include an increased risk of cancer, miscarriage, infertility, and birth defects, along with ongoing water and soil pollution (Karim & Baser, 2022). Furthermore, people suffered multiple traumatic events. According to Taha and Abdurrahman (2020), more than two thirds of the survivors were severely or extremely traumatized, suffering at least 20 traumatic events (including lack of shelter, food or water; confiscation, looting or destruction of personal property; combat situations; witnessing shelling or burning of residential areas; torture; witnessing torture or murder; forced evacuation; etc.). In their study, Taha and Abdurrahman (2020) reported that 86.2% of the survivors studied met the criteria for PTSD.

In addition to individual traumatic experiences, the Anfal campaign and the Halabja chemical attack have shaped Kurdish society for generations, exacerbating existing social and political inequalities (Choman, 2011), leading to collective trauma within the population. The Halabja attack became a significant event in the shared memory and a part of Kurdish identity (Karim & Baser, 2022). The survivors pass on their experiences to subsequent generations, reinforcing memories, and leading to a transgenerational traumatization.

In 2006, after conducting research on the Kurdish people and visiting the Kurdish Region of Iraq (KRI), Prof. Dr. Dr. Jan Ilhan Kizilhan recognized the need for mental health services in the region. He developed the idea of establishing an Institute for Psychotherapy and Psychotraumatology. Despite significant interest from others, there was a lack of funding at the time, so the idea had to be put on hold.

In August 2014, enormous cruelty was once again brought to the KRI, when a terrorist organization, "Islamic State of Iraq and Syria" (ISIS), invaded Iraq and captured provinces in the west and north of the country. Seen as "infidels" by ISIS, they mainly targeted religious minorities, particularly the Yazidi people, who were treated with extreme brutality. Many men were executed, women and children were abducted and raped, and boys turned into child soldiers (Adorjan et al., 2017). These events represented the 74th genocide against the Yazidi people, and have led to massive refugee movements in northern Iraq and Syria. By March 2015, 500,000 Yazidis, predominantly from Sinjar, 190,000 Turkmen Shia from Telafar, 60,000 Shabak Shias, and an equal number of Christians, both from the Ninewa plains, had been displaced (IOM Iraq, 2019). As a consequence of the violence committed by ISIS, and the big influx of refugees, the prevalence of mental disorders rose significantly.

Among Yazidi women who were victims of the 2014 genocide and held captive by ISIS for months, the prevalence for mental disorders were especially high, with 97.9% meeting criteria for PTSD and 88.1% for Major Depression (Kizilhan, Friedl, et al., 2020). The Yazidi people have been subject to repeated genocides and massacres in the past. As a result, current Yazidi victims are experiencing ongoing trauma and feelings of helplessness due to repeated acts of Islamic terrorization (Kizilhan & Noll-Hussong, 2017). They are victims of transgenerational traumatization.

Women abducted by ISIS were subject to brutal sexual violence. In traditional patriarchal societies, being a victim of sexual violence signifies a violation of honor. In collectivist societies like the one in the KRI, these experiences are often concealed to prevent the victims from being excluded from their communities. Yazidi women who were raped by ISIS soldiers face a particularly difficult situation because, according to Yazidi religious beliefs, sexual contact with people outside of their group is not allowed and can lead to being expelled from the community. Thus, the Yazidi women were put in very difficult situations, especially if children were born as a result of the rape. Such women were often not accepted back into their community.

In 2015, the State of Baden-Wuerttemberg launched the "Special Quota Project for vulnerable women and children from northern Iraq", in response to the brutality committed by ISIS. The Special Quota Project poses a unique humanitarian undertaking by the State of Baden-Wuerttemberg in Germany, headed by Dr. Michael Blume. Under this Project, 1,000 women and children were evacuated from the KRI to the state in southern Germany, and 100 more were evacuated to two other German states, Niedersachsen and Schleswig-Holstein.

The Project was aimed at women who had been in the hands of DAESH, were exposed to traumatizing violence, and whose family structures had been broken down through the loss of their male relatives (Junne et al., 2019). Each potential candidate for the project was thoroughly evaluated by a team of three people: (1) Dr Michael Blume, the project head; (2) Prof Dr. Dr. Jan Ilhan Kizilhan, a trauma expert; and (3) an employee in the visa office of the German Consulate General in Erbil. Selection criteria took into account the duration of captivity experienced, the degree of traumatization, medical indications, the collapse of familial support structures, and the prospects for successful treatment in Germany (Junne et al., 2019).

Once they arrived in Germany, the women and children were taken in by more than 20 different communities. They received housing for up to three years, access to medical care, social services, schooling and activities for the children, language classes for the women, as well as psychotherapy in different settings. The families were given the chance to build a future in Germany or to return to their homes in the KRI, if they wished to do so.

An evaluation of the project, conducted by Junne et al. (2019), showed that the majority of the women were satisfied with the Special Quota Project and grateful for the opportunity to build better lives for their children. One of the participants of the project was Nobel Peace Prize laureate Nadia Murad, who publicly shared her story to raise awareness of the brutalities committed by ISIS. The project gave the women a sense of safety and protection, and the ability to take control over their own lives.

One limitation of the Special Quota Project was the bringing these severe trauma survivors to a foreign country with a different culture, language, and traditions. Language barriers and different cultural beliefs about psychological symptoms also posed a barrier for seeking psychotherapeutic help. In addition to the Special Quota Project, it became evident that a broader and more sustainable approach was to help people in the KRI. Interest in Kizilhan's 2006 idea to establish an Institute for Psychotherapy and Psychotraumatology in northern Iraq, aimed at treating traumatized people with culturally sensitive approaches, was rekindled.

As previously described, mental health care is scarce in the KRI. Insufficient health care professionals, a lack of education, difficult access to health services in general, and stigmatization of mental illness all contribute to this. Given the lack of available structures for psychosocial care in the KRI, Prof. Kizilhan's plan to establish an institute for psychotherapy and psychotraumatology, and to train psychotherapists in Kurdistan, promised to be a sustainable solution to improve care in the future. Going beyond the necessary help that MHPSS approaches deliver, the rationale for establishing such an institute was to implement psychotherapy into the health care system and into the education system in the KRI, thus providing a sustainable health care solution. Integrating psychotherapy into institutional structures allows health care workers to collaborate more easily and efficiently. This approach helps reduce stigma associated with mental disorders and makes mental health care more accessible to the general population. Furthermore, integrating the training of psychotherapists into the education system and providing academic-level education for mental health professionals enhances shared knowledge and research, particularly on transcultural aspects of trauma and psychotherapy. This enables local professionals to contribute to international research and become equal academic partners, further advancing their country.

The Institute for Psychotherapy and Psychotraumatology

In 2016, the Institute for Psychotherapy and Psychotraumatology (IPP) was founded at the University of Duhok with support from the state government of Baden-Wuerttemberg in Germany. The establishment of the IPP was coordinated by Prof. Dr. Dr. Jan Ilhan Kizilhan and Prof. Dr. Martin Hautzinger. The IPP officially opened its doors on March 1st, 2017. The organizational structure of the IPP demonstrates the equal collaboration between the KRI and Germany (as shown in Figure 7-1): The IPP is incorporated into the University of Duhok, while German members joined the faculty council for the duration of the project. The directorate of the IPP and the Scientific Advisory Board are made up of members from both northern Iraq and Germany.

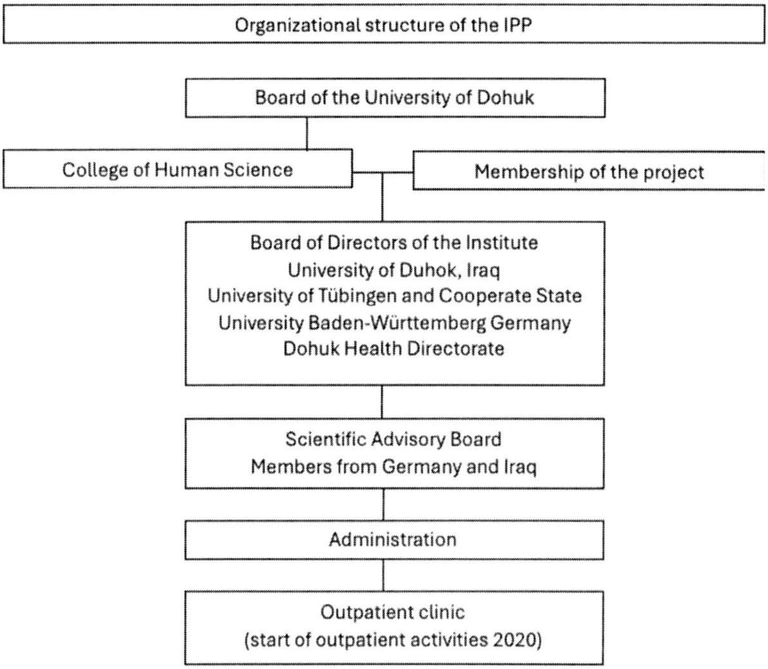

Fig. 7-1 Organizational Structure of the IPP

Tasks of the IPP include researching the basic principles and application of psychotherapy and psychotraumatology, and developing culturally sensitive approaches for use in therapy. A master's program, the *Master of Advanced Studies of Psychotherapy and Psychotraumatology* (MASPP), was developed to train local professionals to become psychotherapists. The IPP supports students to obtain both the MASPP and a license to practice as psychotherapists. Students are further encouraged to pursue doctoral studies at the IPP. Public services provided by the IPP include outpatient psychotherapy in an institute-owned outpatient clinic, and a suicide prevention hotline. The IPP works closely with the University of Duhok, the Ministry of Higher Education, and the Duhok Health Directorate. One of the IPPs goals is to establish a local network of mental health professionals and institutions, including clinicians and researchers.

The IPP and the MASPP are supported and funded by the Ministry of Science, Research and the Arts of Baden-Wuerttemberg, the German Foreign Ministry, and the German Academic Exchange Service. After 2023, the IPP and its activities and responsibilities will be transferred to the

University of Duhok, as stated in a Memorandum of Understanding. This is to ensure the sustainability of the established structures and to avoid dependency on German funds.

Master of Advanced Studies of Psychotherapy and Psychotraumatology (MASPP)

One of the IPP's first challenges was to develop a master's program for training psychotherapists which could keep up with international standards and be integrated into the Iraqi educational system. The program prioritizes: (a) culturally and trauma-informed training, tailored to the local context; (b) sustainability through a team of local professionals who deliver the training; (c) ongoing research to drive continuous improvement and address evolving community needs; and (d) collaborative partnerships with local authorities, government bodies, healthcare services, and academic institutions. The *Master of Advanced Studies of Psychotherapy and Psychotraumatology* (MASPP) is based on the vocational training and examination regulations for licensed psychotherapists in Germany (PsychTh-AprV; see Focus Box 1).

Focus Box 1: Vocational training and examination regulations for licensed psychotherapists in Germany (PsychTh-AprV)

In Germany, *psychotherapist* is a licensed health profession similar to physicians. The vocational training and examination regulations for psychotherapists, which are valid from 1999 until 2020, are based on the Psychotherapists Act (PsychThG) from 1998. During that time, becoming a licensed psychotherapist required a university degree (either a diploma or a master's) in "Psychology". The official job description later became "psychological psychotherapist," distinguishing it from "medical psychotherapist," which referred to physicians trained in psychotherapy.

After the master's degree, postgraduate training was then undertaken at private training institutes. According to PsychTh-AprV, this training comprises a minimum of 4,200 hours and consists of: a practical activity in a psychiatric institution (1,800 hours), theoretical training (600 hours), practical training with outpatient treatment under supervision (600 hours of treatment, 150 hours of supervision), and self-experience, which enables the trainees to reflect on their own therapeutic actions (120 hours). The training concludes with a written and oral state examination.

In 2020, the regulations for psychotherapist training changed, and a university degree in "Psychotherapy" was introduced. The contents of the training remain the same as stated in PsychTh-AprV.

The German training was adapted to the official *Master Study Regulations at Public Universities in the Kurdistan Region,* as set out by the Ministry of Higher Education and Scientific Research. It was expanded to include a focus on trauma therapy as well as culturally sensitive approaches. One necessary change was shortening the training period from the three years typical of German education, to the two-year standard for master's studies in the KRI. This was resolved by adding a one-year preparatory phase to the two-year master's program. Furthermore, the number and type of exams and other assessments had to be adapted to be comparable to other master's programs at Kurdish universities.

To ensure inclusion of all necessary teaching content, the MASPP consists of a preparatory year and a two-year master's program, which concludes with a master's thesis and defense. The focus of the one-year preparation phase is the acquisition of basic knowledge about concepts of cognitive-behavioral therapy (CBT). It also includes English classes. At the end of the preparation year, students must pass a language skills exam in order to continue the program. The two-year master's program aims to teach more specialized knowledge regarding diagnostics and treatment of psychological disorders. See Table 7-1 for an overview of the subjects taught in the two-year master's program.

Table 7-1 Subjects of the Two-year Master's Program

First Year	Second Year
Introduction and refreshment of psychology, psychotherapy, and psychotraumatology	Theories of Holistic Psychotherapy
Psychopathology	Assessments
Group Dynamics	Trauma and treatment of trauma
Developmental Psychology Across the Lifespan	Clinical Practice and Supervision II: Clinical Setting
Clinical Skills	Master's thesis
Psychological Disorders ICD 10 (F10-90)	6 Case Reports
Psychology of Culture and Identity: Power, Privilege and Oppression	
Quantitative and Qualitative Research Methods	

Professional Psychology and Psychotherapy	
Theories of Psychotherapy	
Psychological Trauma and Post-Trauma Therapy	
Disaster Mental Health and Community Crisis Intervention	
Trauma in the Lives of Children and Adolescents	
Clinical Practice and Supervision I: Clinical Setting	

The MASPP provides a broad understanding of the theoretical principles and practical implementation of psychotherapy and psychotraumatology, which are necessary for safe and effective clinical and scientific work. The training enables graduates to practice as highly qualified psychotherapists with a specialization in psychotraumatology. It prepares them to work both within the health care system and in the academic field. Key factors guiding the development of the program were that the training should be grounded in evidence-based international standards and be culturally and trauma sensitive. A number of international experts agreed to function as lecturers in the first cohorts of the MASPP. To ensure sustainability of the program, a core group of graduates are being trained as local lecturers to ensure continued training for further students.

The curriculum for the master's program was developed under the leadership of Prof. Dr. Martin Hautzinger. Since the German psychotherapist training starts after the master's degree, and thus assumes a higher level of knowledge, some content on the basics of mental illness and research methods had to be added to the curriculum. Due to the high number of traumatized people in the KRI, the German curriculum was extended to include a focus on psychotraumatology. Trauma therapeutic treatment approaches were prioritized at the beginning of the curriculum and different approaches were taught in depth. The curriculum also focuses on addressing cross-cultural differences and teaching culturally-sensitive treatment approaches. Religious and cultural beliefs influence the perception and interpretation of psychological symptomatology and therefore must be considered in treatment (Kizilhan, 2014). In particular, potential interreligious conflicts, such as those found in the KRI, should be considered. For example, as a result of the brutality used by ISIS against those of other faiths, patients who are Yazidi may express mistrust of Muslim therapists (Wolf et al., 2019). Moreover, in traditional, collectivist societies, relationships within the family and the well-being of the entire social fabric play a greater role than individual needs. Therapeutic approaches taught in Germany are oriented to Western values, which mainly focus on the well-being of the individual client, and therefore need to be adapted.

In line with PsychTh-AprV (see Infobox 1), psychotherapist training in Germany consists of theoretical and practical elements. Accordingly, the MASPP includes lectures, seminars, experiential learning in small and large groups, small group supervision and clinical placements, as well as individual tutorials. Students are encouraged to actively engage in all the components of the training. The parallel integration of theoretical, practical, and self-reflective modules under supervision enables a deep understanding of psychotherapy and therapeutic impact factors. However, cultural differences need to be taken into account regarding the use of didactic methods. For example, because of a much more hierarchical instruction style in Iraqi teaching, students are not accustomed to class discussions where they must stand out and apply critical thinking (Mohammed-Marzouk, 2012). Cultural differences must also be reflected upon with students in the context of culturally sensitive clinical supervision and personal experience sessions (Wolf et al., 2019).

Figure 7-2 shows the detailed sequence of the theoretical and practical components over the course of the program. In accordance with the German psychotherapist training, the individual elements of the MASPP are:

- Theoretical training (600 units of 45 minutes)
- Practical experience in psychiatric institutions, refugee camps, clinics (1800 units of 60 minutes)
- Treatment of outpatients with various mental disorders (600 units of 50 minutes)
- Clinical supervision (150 units of 50 minutes)
- Personal experience, which encompasses reflecting one's own person and experiencing therapy methods in the client role (120 units of 50 minutes)
- Independent knowledge acquisition by means of eLearning modules (see chapter XX; 120 units of 45 minutes), homework (370 units of 45 minutes) and treatment documentation (440 units of 45 minutes)

Theoretical training modules take place as two-week block courses in the IPP at the University of Duhok. These training blocks include theoretical seminars, study groups, supervision/intervision groups, and personal experience reflection sessions (see Focus Box 2).

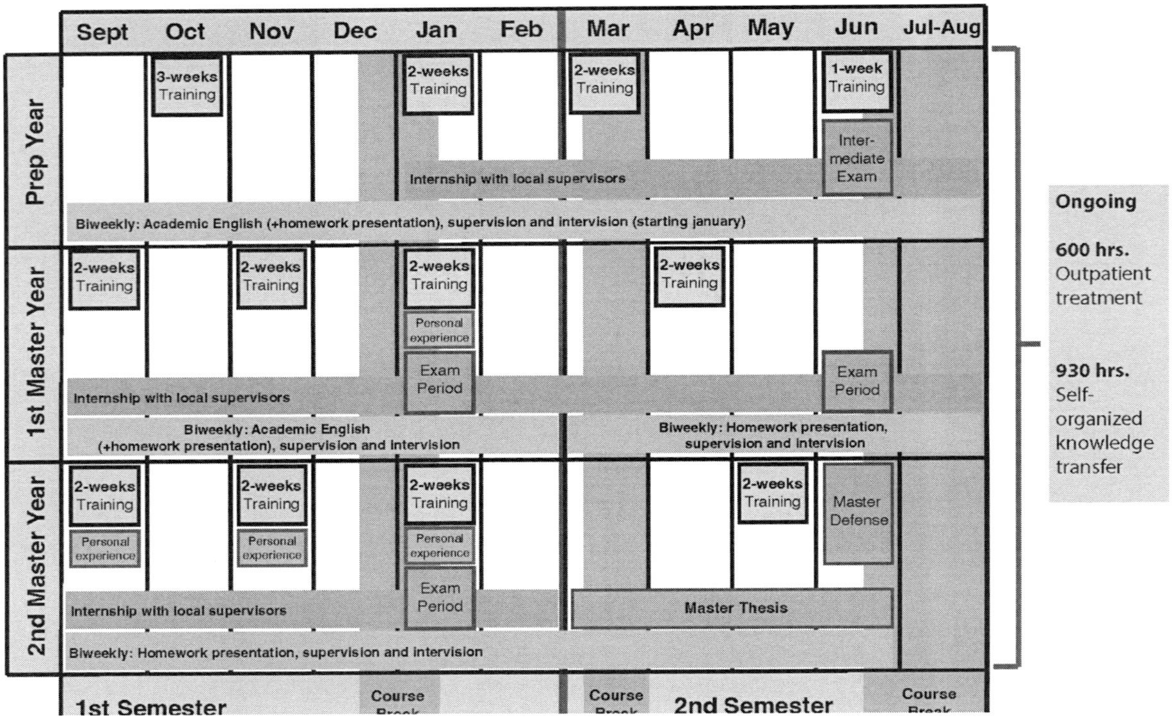

Fig 7-2 Components of the Master's Program

Focus Box 2: Supervision, Intervision, and Self-Experience

Supervision

The nature and role of supervision is used to give support/guidance for dealing with any difficulties/obstacles experienced by the client and therapist during therapy sessions. The supervision is provided in one-to-one monthly sessions by the IPP, as well as two-hour group sessions each month. The goal of supervision is to encourage the supervisee to reflect on their own actions and to improve their professional skills. Possible exposure to secondary traumatic symptoms can also be addressed and reviewed as part of supervision, in order to prevent chronification. Supervision can also include case presentations with specific questions. Supervision is led by an experienced psychotherapist.

Intervision

Intervision refers to the discussion and processing of difficulties in the therapy process in small groups of colleagues. Using set instructions, Intervision is led by the participants themselves and is recorded. It serves to encourage self-reflection about professional and personal issues related to psychotherapy.

Self-Experience

Self-experience can take place in groups or in individual settings. The goal is to reflect on one's own life history, inner beliefs, and therapeutic attitude. The therapist can slip into the role of their clients and experience therapy methods firsthand. Self-experience helps to develop one's own ability to reflect and to be able to distinguish one's own issues from those of the client.

Students are encouraged to start their practical activities right at the beginning of the program and complete them in parallel with the theoretical block seminars. The practical activities are performed in Azadi Hospital in Duhok or in one of the NGOs that are usually active in the refugee camps. The students work in a team environment within the respective NGO and under the guidance of the NGO itself. Some of the NGOs provide supervision, otherwise students are supervised by specialized supervisors at the IPP, or online by international supervisors. At the end of the program, students must write and orally defend a master's thesis. The thesis consists of six case reports and a theoretical-scientific component.

A prerequisite for participation in the MASPP is the completion of a bachelor's degree in psychology, medicine, or social work. Applicants must participate in a special selection seminar with one-on-one interviews regarding scientific and therapeutic proficiency. As the main teaching language is English throughout the whole program, participants have to prove their proficiency in the English language after being accepted and before beginning the master's program. If applicants do not fulfil the requirements for English language, they can enhance their language skills over the period of the preparation year. Participation in the program is free of charge since it has been covered by the Ministry of Science, Research and the Arts of Baden-Wuerttemberg, the German Foreign Ministry, and the German Academic Exchange Service, to date.

The first group of students started the program in February 2017 and, of the original 30 students, 28 successfully completed the master's program in April 2020. Out of the second cohort, which started in October 2018, 21 out of 24 students graduated in November 2021. The third cohort of 25 students began the preparatory year in October 2020 and 20 students completed the master's program in fall 2023. A fourth cohort of 28 students started training in May 2023 and will graduate in fall 2026.

e-Learning

The use of educational technology to support teaching and learning at the IPP played an important role from the outset of the project. A digital learning environment on the platform “Moodle” (https://moodle.com/) was created to facilitate communication between German, international, and Kurdish administrators, lecturers, and students. As both the Baden-Wuerttemberg Cooperative State University and the University of Duhok were already using Moodle, the choice of platform was easy to make. The use of e-Learning tools was considered obvious because they are now a standard part of education at universities worldwide. In addition, they facilitate the international communication necessary for the implementation of the MASPP. Against the backdrop of limited security in a post-conflict region, and the ongoing threat of new conflicts, the digital learning environment promises the possibility to continue working with each other from home. This certainly proved useful in the face of the COVID-19 pandemic. Using Moodle was also helpful for sustainability as Moodle courses created for a particular student cohort could be used for structuring courses for subsequent student cohorts. It also becomes easy to create a pool of teaching and learning materials for subsequent cohorts by collecting them in the digital learning platform.

Together, German and local Kurdish staff developed e-Learning content specifically designed for the project. This included the development of two interactive Moodle courses: the "eTrauma Workbook," for learning about diagnosing and treating trauma related disorders, and "Scientific Methods," for learning about conducting scientific research and publishing scientific articles. Furthermore, the platform facilitates independent study, the provision of study materials and learning goals from international and local lecturers, and the uploading of homework and study progress by students. In addition, access to international professional online journals and books has been provided through the University of Tuebingen's library, via VPN.

"Training-of-Trainers" Program

Many international experts in psychotherapy and psychotraumatology were interested in the project and joined the IPP as lecturers for the first cohort of the master's program starting in 2017. They agreed to travel to Duhok a few times to give their lectures. The students of the IPP benefited a lot from this support and the knowledge shared by international researchers and clinicians.

The goal, however, was to ensure sustainability in the training of psychotherapists, by training local stakeholders that would continue to teach students at the IPP. Hence, a "training-of-trainers" (TOT) approach was planned from the outset. Selected students from the first cohorts (so far, five students from the first cohort and two students from the second cohort) were trained as lecturers and assumed increasing responsibility for teaching and administrative activities at the IPP while completing their master's. During this time, they functioned as co-lecturers, assisting the international experts with teaching and supervision of the following cohort. This way, they were able to gain first-hand practical experience in education under the supervision of an international lecturer, before taking over teaching. The students selected for the TOT-program took part in additional training courses on study organization, management, and didactics. By implementing this gradual approach, they were able to take over more and more key components of the project. Figure 7-3 illustrates the required steps that local lecturers are required to take to assume responsibility of the project. In the long-term, this approach is thought to help graduates of the IPP develop their skills further, become leaders and organizers on the project, and thus help advance psychotherapy in their own country. Many of the co-lecturers are pursuing their doctoral studies at the same time, sometimes in close collaboration with the international lecturers they met at the IPP.

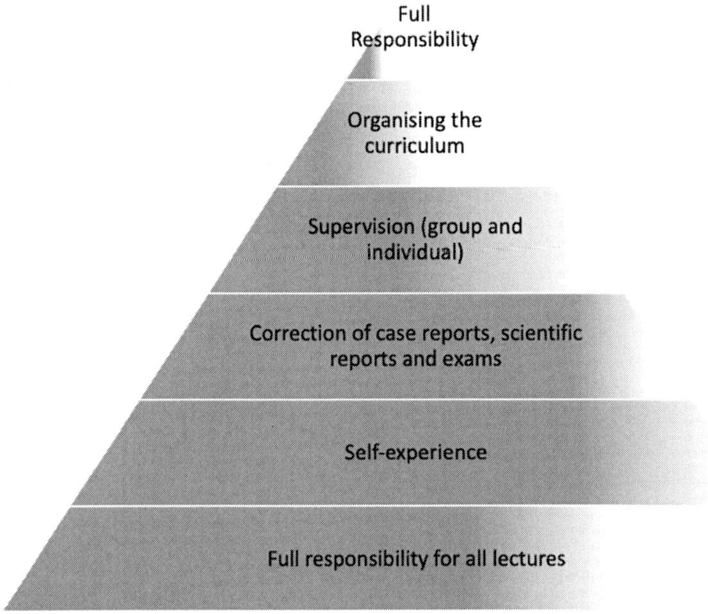

Fig. 7-3 Required Steps for Local Lecturers to Assume Full Responsibility (Kornwachs et al., 2024)
Note. Green color indicates the estimated degree of progress.

The IPP During the Pandemic

In March 2020, the World Health Organization (WHO) declared the outbreak of the coronavirus disease 2019 (COVID -19) global pandemic (World Health Organization, 2020). The severity of the outbreak led many countries to declare it as a public health emergency. Many countries consequently implemented far-reaching measures to stop its spread, such as social distancing rules, travel restrictions, emergency response procedures, and lockdowns. The Kurdistan Region of Iraq (KRI) was also affected by the spread of the virus. By the end of 2020, there were roughly 103,000 confirmed cases of COVID-19 infections in the KRI. By the end of 2021, this number was approximately 380,500 cases (Kurdistan Regional Government, 2023). The Kurdistan Regional Government (KRG) reacted with several measures to control the spread of the virus. These included raising awareness, closing schools and universities between February 2020 and September 2020, and cancellation of public gatherings such as Friday prayers, church gatherings, funerals, and weddings. A curfew was enforced from March to June 2020, followed by a partial curfew until August 2020. Additionally, mandatory quarantine was required for travelers entering the country, along with social distancing and disinfection principles (Hussein et al., 2020; Kurdistan Regional Government, 2023).

The already overwhelmed healthcare system in the KRI suffered from a lack of equipment and personnel. A dire financial situation further contributed to a surge in COVID-19-cases (Shehata et al., 2021). The refugee camps in the region were particularly affected. There were outbreaks of COVID-19 in the camps, which were difficult to control. Isolation measures in the camps burdened the residents, as access to essential and emergency services was hindered by COVID-19 restrictions (Shehata et al., 2021).

The IPP was also affected by the pandemic and the restrictions that came with it. When international travel was suspended, experts, lecturers, and project staff from outside the KRI were not able to come to the IPP. Meetings between the project leaders from Germany and other project staff were not possible. Meetings between the trauma network partners also could not be held. As universities were closed, lectures had to be canceled.

Like in many parts of the world, teaching and meetings were moved online. The existing e-Learning environment on the platform "Moodle" proved to be particularly helpful and eased the conversion process. Exchange of information and documents was made very easy through the platform. Students were able to work remotely and had access to all necessary materials at any time. International experts were able to hold their lectures from home via online meetings, and supervision and personal experience seminars were also conducted online. For events that could not be held online easily, the Training the Trainer (TOT) program participants (students that were being trained to take over teaching responsibilities at a later point) were asked to step in. This was the case for personal experience seminars. Two TOTs conducted the seminars while receiving daily online supervision from German experts. Thus, the TOTs assumed teaching responsibilities much sooner than originally planned.

All in all, the measures taken to deal with the restrictions of the pandemic were successful and the IPP's activities continued smoothly. The e-Learning environment, which was originally set up in case of renewed conflicts in the area, proved to be very useful in this situation. A minor criticism from the lecturers was that students often attended the lectures on their cell phones, while on the move, and were therefore not fully engaged in the subject matter. The early involvement of the TOT participants, on the other hand, was rated very positively. At the beginning, there were concerns as to whether they would be up to the task if they were thrown in at the deep end. In retrospect, however, the engagement and performance of the TOT participants was evaluated very positively. Many of the international experts and project staff recommended that, in hindsight, the TOT participants should have been involved as early as possible in the process of setting up a project like the IPP.

The operations of the German Clinic for Psychotherapy, which opened in 2021, remained largely unaffected by the events of the pandemic. At the time of the opening, the first study group had already completed their program, and therapies could proceed without restrictions. Weekly intervisions and supervisions were conducted, supplemented by two additional online supervisions per month from Germany.

Networking

In collaboration with the Ministry of Health in Duhok, the German Agency for International Cooperation GmbH (Deutsche Gesellschaft für Internationale Zusammenarbeit GmbH, GIZ) and several NGOs, the IPP has been working on establishing a trauma network since 2018. The goal is to establish a long-term and stable connection between medical, psychological, and nursing professionals, as well as academics and researchers, working in the care of extremely traumatized people. To start, the network has focused its work on the Duhok governorate, aiming to expand its reach across all of the KRI in the future.

As a first step, the trauma network wants to raise awareness for mental illness, psychotrauma, and trauma sequelae in the population by offering seminars, training, congresses, and publications of work. Further, an interdisciplinary network in the scientific and clinical community is being built up to develop new therapy approaches, such as culturally-sensitive methods and techniques. By improving connections between existing services (e.g., counseling services, institutions, therapists, crisis interventions services, and NGOs), and helping them to cooperate with each other, better and faster access to the necessary help can be provided for the population. Further goals include regular network meetings for information sharing and training seminars, creation of a scientific network, genocide and peace research, as well as reconciliation and memory work dealing with genocide.

As a way to draw international attention to the KRI, and to create international and local connections, the IPP has organized three international conferences. The First International Conference on Genocide and Trauma took place in May 2018. More than 300 experts from 16 countries, and survivors of genocide from Rwanda, Cambodia, Nepal, Guatemala, and Bosnia, took part in the conference and shared their experiences on how to deal with trauma and genocide. Experts from Harvard and New York joined the conference as well. Topics of the conference included trauma associated mental disorders, their treatment in adults and children, as well as discussions about "Mental Health and Psychosocial Support" (MHPSS) approaches. Specifics of gender and trauma were discussed, as well as the prevention and intervention of collective violence. Next to the international experts, students of the IPP shared their experiences from the KRI.

In June 2019, the second international conference, titled "East meets West," focused on the exchange of global and local methods in psychosocial work, psychotherapy, and psychotraumatology between Middle Eastern and Western countries. Researchers and clinicians from the Middle East, Europe, the USA, and Africa discussed several topics, including mental disorders and their treatment, trauma following genocide and mass violence, mass trauma, prevention of collective violence, reconciliation and reparation, and trauma in children and ethnic/religious minorities. More than 300 participants learned from 46 speakers, from 11 countries, about different treatment methods developed in the Western world. They learned about how these Western treatment methods can help in other cultures, as well as which regional differences need to be taken into account when providing support.

A third international conference on "Psychotherapy in Conflict and Post- Conflict Regions" took place in November 2022. It provided a stage to discuss different perspectives on psychosocial support and psychotherapy, and the integration of interventions with adults, children, and youth. Mental health issues of refugees and internally displaces persons (IDPs) posed an important topic of the conference, as well as aspects of transgenerational trauma. Furthermore, the experts from Europe and the Middle East discussed interdisciplinary interventions in war, torture, and flight. The IPP was able to use this conference to showcase its current work and future plans.

Research Activities

Establishing a psychotherapy institute in conflict and post-conflict regions not only serves the immediate need for mental health support but also presents a unique opportunity for impactful research and international collaboration. Therefore, another key focus of the IPP was to facilitate research activities. By fostering international scientific connections, the IPP opened avenues for cross-cultural collaboration and knowledge exchange. Connecting with global researchers and institutions provided access to a broader spectrum of theories, methodologies, and best practices in psychotherapy. The linguistic diversity of the local graduates was an especially valuable resource for conducting research that delves into the intricacies of culturally-specific therapeutic needs and approaches. The availability of a diverse patient population within the IPP's network also presented an opportunity for meaningful research.

Perceived Injustice Questionnaire

An example of a research activity which has taken place at the IPP is the development of the Perceived Injustice Questionnaire (PIQ). In response to the intricate relationship between mental disorders and perceived injustice among survivors of war and displacement, the development of the 24-item Perceived Injustice Questionnaire (PIQ, see Appendix A) was initiated (Neumann et al., 2021). Initially validated within a cohort of MASPP students, the PIQ displayed a four-factor structure and demonstrated satisfactory reliability. Aligning with the objective of creating a transculturally applicable tool, the PIQ underwent translation into Ukrainian. It has been established that the Ukrainian version exhibits excellent overall reliability. Moreover, the PIQ demonstrates strong correlations with post-traumatic stress disorder (PTSD) symptoms, as well as moderate associations with symptoms of depression and generalized anxiety disorder. Importantly, the Ukrainian version of the PIQ predicted symptoms of PTSD, depression, and generalized anxiety disorder beyond exposure to potentially traumatic life events (paper currently under review for publication).

Other Research Projects

In addition to research on injustice perceptions, the IPP has contributed to a total of 32 papers, addressing diverse focal points within the broader context of conflict and post-conflict regions.

A substantial body of work has been dedicated to the exploration of psychological impacts of genocide and transgenerational trauma (e.g., Kizilhan et al., 2023; Kizilhan et al., 2021). Another focus has centered on the unique psychological vulnerability of women in the context of war and terror, along with the consequences of sexual violence (e.g., Kizilhan,

Steger, et al., 2020). Additionally, various publications have emerged related to education and the establishment of psychotherapeutic services (e.g., Beckmann et al., 2022; Steger & Kizilhan, 2022; Wolf et al., 2019), as well as specific therapeutical interventions (e.g., Kizilhan, 2019; Kizilhan & Wenzel, 2020), in the context of conflict and post-conflict regions. Work on secondary trauma among healthcare professionals (Denkinger et al., 2018; Kizilhan, 2020) and socio-psychological aspects of Islamized terror (Kizilhan, 2018; Kizilhan & Steger, 2021) have also been produced. A publication list of these papers can be found in the appendices (see Appendix B). The diverse range of research reflects a commitment to addressing multifaceted aspects of psychotraumatology, fostering a holistic approach to the mental well-being of individuals in conflict-affected areas. In essence, the research activities stemming from the establishment of the IPP not only contributed to the global body of knowledge in clinical psychology, psychotraumatology, and the psychological effects of war, violence, and displacement, but also foster a deeper understanding of local cultures and languages. This dual approach enables the IPP to play a pivotal role in advancing both international and regional perspectives in the field of psychotherapy.

Emergency Suicide Prevention Hotline

Background

Several studies have highlighted elevated rates of suicidal ideation, suicide attempts, and completed suicide within refugee populations (Akinyemi et al., 2015; Hermans et al., 2017; Kim et al., 2007; Rahman & Hafeez, 2003; Tay et al., 2019). Suicidal ideation is particularly prevalent among those residing in refugee camps, representing one of the most common mental health challenges (Hermans et al., 2017; Kizilhan et al., 2023). Particularly concerning is a striking example among Yazidi women who have previously experienced enslavement. This specific group not only grapples with an elevated prevalence of psychological stress (97.1%), PTSD (90.6%), depression (36.7%), and general anxiety symptoms (37.4%), but also exhibits an increased incidence of suicidal ideation (38.1%) (Kizilhan et al., 2023; Taha & Slewa-Younan, 2020). Among Yazidis in Northern Iraq, those primarily from the Sinjar region who directly experienced the 2014 ISIS attack exhibit the highest levels of vulnerability to suicidal thoughts. This contrasts with those from the less affected Duhok region (Kizilhan et al., 2023). Given suicide is often stigmatized in these societies, leading to discrimination and exclusion (Jäger et al., 2019), the reported data raises significant concerns and a call for action.

Project Description

One of the services offered by the IPP, since March 2021, is an Emergency Suicide Prevention Hotline for everyone in the Duhok governorate, including refugee and IDP camps. The hotline is intended for people with suicidal thoughts or for people that know someone showing signs of being suicidal. The hotline can be reached 24 hours a day and is free to call. Four psychotherapists working in shifts cover the hotline and confidentiality is ensured. The attending psychotherapists listen and talk with the caller to help stabilize them. They then refer them to the IPP clinic, the German Clinic for Psychotherapy (described later), or to the psychiatric department at Azadi hospital in Duhok. In emergency cases, the psychotherapists talk to family members of the caller. The impact of the hotline has been recorded, with the data for 2023 shown in Figure 7-4.

Total number of calls	Actual suicide calls	Cases with psychological problems	Information seeking calls	Referrals to clinic/ other service providers	Follow up calls
242	49	53	138	60	57

Fig. 7-4 Case Numbers of Emergency Suicide Prevention Hotline for 2023

Additionally, the Suicide Prevention Hotline team offers information events in schools, government agencies, and refugee camps, to educate people about mental illness and suicide. The team also distributes brochures among the general population to create awareness about suicide and to spread knowledge about how to help someone with suicidal thoughts.

Infrastructure

Team members are recruited through IPP staff and receive additional training in the assessment of suicidality. Presently, three out of the four psychotherapists are graduates of the MASPP. The team is proficient in Kurdish, Kurmanji, and Sorani. Members work remotely from home and receive compensation from German donors (Caritas International,

Schwaebische Zeitung, and Eric Gustav-Adler Foundation). Telephone expenses are covered by IPP project funds.

Publicity

Currently, flyers and posters are used to raise awareness about the hotline (see Appendix C). There are upcoming plans to enhance visibility of the hotline through the establishment of a dedicated website and presence on social media platforms. The IT department at the University of Duhok is actively supporting the hotline in these initiatives.

German Clinic for Psychotherapy

In February 2021, the IPP established the "German Clinic for Psychotherapy", a German-style outpatient clinic (see Appendix D). In Germany, outpatient clinics are often part of hospitals and university clinics, where they are designed to combine clinical care, teaching, and research.

The goal of the "German Clinic for Psychotherapy" is to offer assessment and diagnosis of psychological and psychosomatic problems, as well as outpatient psychotherapeutic treatment based on cognitive behavioral therapy. There are currently eight graduates of the IPP working at the clinic as psychotherapists, treating people from refugee camps as well as from the city of Duhok. One physician is supporting the psychotherapists with medical assessments. The clinic is equipped with a small reception room and three rooms for therapy sessions. It contains a small library with textbooks and psychological testing materials for assessments and diagnostics.

The treatment is free for patients because high fees are a typical barrier to seeking help (besides stigma). To further reduce fears and stigma, a local community member with similar linguistic and ethnic (Yazidi) background has been hired as a first contact to explain services and answer questions about psychotherapy. After a first screening with a psychotherapist, clients are either referred to more suited services or, if indeed in need of psychotherapy, registered as clinic clients. Clients will then receive a medical and a psychiatric consultation, and undergo a thorough psychotherapy intake, which includes an intake interview and diagnostic measures. Before treatment begins, the diagnosis and treatment plan are determined through a case discussion between the therapist, the Head of the clinic, and either the medical doctor or psychiatrist. If a psychological disorder is diagnosed, psychotherapy treatment will begin, and psychiatric treatment will be provided if needed.

In 2023, 167 patients received 1,385 sessions at the German Clinic for Psychotherapy, with an average number of 8 sessions per patient. The main diagnoses included major depressive disorder, anxiety disorders, obsessive compulsive disorders, and PTSD.

In the future, research will also be carried out in the German Clinic for Psychotherapy. This research will continuously contribute to expanding knowledge about the causes, maintenance, and modifiability of mental problems or illnesses. This knowledge will be directly incorporated into the therapy services offered by the German Clinic, aiming to ensure a high standard of quality in diagnosis, counseling, and therapy. The German Clinic will also support students of the MASPP with their training and provide internship positions.

Clinic in Sinjar

The majority of refugees living in the camps in the Duhok province come from the Shingal area of the Duhok province. They intend to return to their settlement areas in the short- and long-term. This agreement was reached by the governments of Baghdad and Erbil with the support of the UN in December 2020. Currently, approximately 130,000 to 150,000 people reside in the Shingal area, where the healthcare infrastructure is nearly non-existent due to the destruction of cities and villages. Due to a significant number of returnees, both the international community and the German Ministry of Development are focused on assisting in the reconstruction of the devastated areas and providing people with the option of returning, despite ongoing political challenges. Several international NGOs operate in locations like Khane Sor and Sinune, not far from the largest city, Sinjar.

To support health care in this particular region, the German Clinic for Psychotherapy initiated the establishment of a branch in Sinjar in 2021 (see Appendix E). The aim of this branch is to provide on-site psychotherapeutic treatment for the local population. Similar to the main outpatient clinic, the clinic in Sinjar primarily assists individuals who have experienced psychological distress due to displacement and war. The branch is supervised and evaluated by the IPP. In 2023, 82 patients received 826 sessions at the Sinjar Clinic, with an average number of 10 sessions per patient.

For security reasons, the clinic had to be relocated to one of the refugee camps in Sinune, which is 20 kilometers from Sinjar. This facility now caters to the returnees from Sinjar in 2021 and 2022 (approximately 50,000 refugees) and provides necessary treatment and support. When conditions permit, the clinic will reopen in Sinjar. For now, initial discussions regarding the premises in Sinune have taken place. Four psychotherapists originally from Sinjar will migrate there with the refugees and operate the clinic in collaboration with the IPP. The branch is set to commence operations in 2024.

Outlook: Challenges in Handing Over Responsibilities

The idea to establish an Institute for Psychotherapy and Psychotraumatology (IPP), and to train psychotherapists in northern Iraq, began in 2006. Ten years later, in 2016, the IPP first opened its doors. Since then, a total of 69 psychotherapists have graduated from the master's program and are treating patients in the KRI. Most of them are working in high positions in local or international NGOs. In addition, seven students have been "trained as trainers," taking on teaching responsibilities and administrative tasks at the IPP, thus helping to ensure its future. Two outpatient psychotherapy clinics belong to the IPP, one in Duhok and one in Sinjar, and are giving the population access to psychotherapy. In short, the training of psychotherapists and the integration of psychotherapeutic care into the health care system has commenced successfully.

However, the challenges continue. The fourth cohort of students started training in 2023 and will be graduating in March 2026. At the same time, the Baden-Wuerttemberg Cooperative State University and the University of Duhok are working towards transferring the IPP and all its activities completely to the University of Duhok. Since its beginning, the project was funded by the Ministry of Science, Research and the Arts of Baden-Wuerttemberg, the German Foreign Ministry, and the German Academic Exchange Service. Administrative tasks as well as the organization of the curriculum were in German hands, and lecturers were mostly German or international experts in their respective fields. As shown in the organizational structure of the IPP in Figure 1, the main positions are occupied by Kurdish and German members. Now it is time to transfer all administrative activities, teaching, and financial responsibilities from Germany to the University of Duhok in order to ensure sustainability. The first TOT participants, who are local graduates of the IPP trained to become lecturers, are already taking over more and more tasks. They are expected to fully take over teaching at IPP starting in March 2026. Sustainability can only be ensured if the University of Duhok takes over the financial responsibility for the IPP.

Legal Recognition

Close cooperation with the Ministry of Higher Education and the Health Directorate of the KRG plays a central role in the inclusion of psychotherapy into the health care system. As previously described, there is a lack of psychotherapy expertise in health care education in northern Iraq. Psychotherapists are not distinguished from other mental health professionals and so far, psychotherapy is not governed by legislation. Hence, an important next step is to legally establish the profession of psychotherapist. This will give local professionals the recognition they deserve, including financial recognition, and will help make psychotherapy more distinguishable from other health professions. The aim is to introduce a draft law that protects the profession of psychotherapy. Up until now, the vocational training regulations of the MASPP contain a clause that students must stay and work in the country for four years after completing the program. To make working in the country more attractive for IPP graduates, working conditions and recognition of their profession must improve.

Navigating Hierarchical Challenges

The regional university system is highly hierarchical, often hindering practical solutions and favorable working conditions. Higher-ranked decision-makers prioritize maintaining their positions and bureaucratic barriers, limiting the freedom of research and student opportunities. Despite some political goodwill, hierarchical resistance can affect even high-quality ideas. This rigid structure conflicts with modern psychotherapy principles, where equality between therapist and beneficiary is key. In Kurdish culture, age, gender, and position heavily influence perceived authority, challenging younger local lecturers' acceptance. To address this, it is essential to support local staff while respecting existing structures. International experts should visibly endorse local lecturers, enhancing their credibility and fostering respect among students and university figures. Simultaneously, a balance must be struck by involving key hierarchical figures in organizational matters, to meet their need for control, without allowing bureaucratic micromanagement to stifle the project. This dual approach helps integrate modern practices while acknowledging and navigating traditional hierarchies.

Awareness and Professional Representation

The profession of psychotherapist is still not well known in the KRI. The treatment of mental disorders currently lies in the hands of psychiatrists, who regard themselves as the only experts and assert exclusive decision-making authority over the care of patients. To become equal partners in the treatment of patients, the extensive training and expertise of psychotherapists must be promoted and acknowledged. An association for psychotherapists needs to be founded to raise awareness about their profession and to achieve representation of their interests in society and government.

Collaborating with Psychiatrists

Initially, the program faced resistance from local psychiatrists, who undermined the new profession's authority. With the project's growing reputation and the valuable work of the graduates, this issue has improved. Including psychiatrists in the project as lecturers and examiners has enhanced the curriculum and fostered trust in psychotherapy. This collaboration serves as a model for future cooperation between psychiatry and psychotherapy, both academically and in practical settings.

Expanding Educational Pathways

Psychotherapy is not yet established as part of the education system in the KRI. In 2021, only the University of Koya offered a master's degree in clinical psychology. To further ensure the qualification of psychotherapists, ideas are being developed to establish a College of Psychology at the University of Duhok and to improve the teaching curriculum of the Bachelor of Psychology as a foundation for the MASPP. Hopefully the MASPP can serve as a model for other universities in the country.

Challenges in Transcultural Supervision

In supervision, MASPP students often felt tested, and focused on showcasing positive progress rather than discussing challenges openly. This may stem from the hierarchical structure of academia and cultural emphasis on oral exams. Supervisors must clarify that supervision isn't an exam and create an error-tolerant, benevolent environment. They should help students critically reflect on therapy processes and acknowledge small steps as therapeutic progress. Supervision also involves supporting students emotionally and addressing therapist self-care to build resilience in facing challenging situations.

Navigating Cultural and Ethical Challenges

Local students and lecturers face the complex task of integrating cultural traditions with modern psychotherapy ethics. For instance, the perception of homosexuality as a disorder conflicts with contemporary therapeutic principles, leading to dilemmas in treatment planning. Clients' reservations regarding therapist attributes underscore the importance of cultural understanding and demythologization. Therapists must balance traditional healing beliefs with evidence-based practices, navigating cultural norms to build trustful relationships. Here, supervisors are crucial for guiding therapists in addressing conflicts without immediate solutions, emphasizing the value of incremental progress and non-judgmental support in therapy sessions.

In summary, the project has successfully initiated psychotherapist training and integrated psychotherapy into northern Iraq's healthcare system. The next steps involve transferring all responsibilities to the University of Duhok, ensuring financial sustainability, and gaining legal recognition for psychotherapists. Balancing support for local staff while respecting hierarchical structures will be crucial. Continued collaboration with local psychiatrists, local authorities, and enhancements in education will further solidify psychotherapy's role in the region.

References

Adorjan, K., Odenwald, M., Kizilhan, J., Pogarell, O., Mulugeta, S., Ndetei, D., Osman, A., Hautzinger, M., Wolf, S., & Othman, M. (2017). Psychiatrische Versorgung von Flüchtlingen in Afrika und dem Nahen Osten. *Der Nervenarzt*, *88*(9).

Akinyemi, O., Atilola, O., & Soyannwo, T. (2015). Suicidal ideation: Are refugees more at risk compared to host population? Findings from a preliminary assessment in a refugee community in Nigeria. *Asian journal of psychiatry*, *18*, 81-85.

Beckmann, J., Wenzel, T., Hautzinger, M., & Kizilhan, J. I. (2022). Training of psychotherapists in post-conflict regions: A Community case study in the Kurdistan Region of Iraq [Community Case Study]. *Frontiers in Psychiatry*, *13*. https://doi.org/10.3389/fpsyt.2022.947903

Black, G. (1993). *Genocide in Iraq: the Anfal campaign against the Kurds*. Human Rights Watch.

Bolton, P., Michalopoulos, L., Ahmed, A. M. A., Murray, L. K., & Bass, J. (2013). The mental health and psychosocial problems of survivors of torture and genocide in Kurdistan, Northern Iraq: a brief qualitative study. *Torture*, *23*(1), 1-14.

Choman, H. (2011). *Gendered experiences of genocide: Anfal survivors in Kurdistan-Iraq*. Ashgate Publishing.

Denkinger, J. K., Windthorst, P., Rometsch-Ogioun El Sount, C., Blume, M., Sedik, H., Kizilhan, J. I., Gibbons, N., Pham, P., Hillebrecht, J., & Ateia, N. (2018). Secondary traumatization in caregivers working with women and children who suffered extreme violence by the "islamic state". *Frontiers in Psychiatry*, *9*, 234.

Hermans, M. P., Kooistra, J., Cannegieter, S. C., Rosendaal, F. R., Mook-Kanamori, D. O., & Nemeth, B. (2017). Healthcare and disease burden among refugees in long-stay refugee camps at Lesbos, Greece. *European journal of epidemiology*, *32*, 851-854.

Hussein, N. R., Naqid, I. A., Saleem, Z. S. M., Musa, D. H., & Ibrahim, N. (2020). The impact of breaching lockdown on the spread of COVID-19 in Kurdistan region, Iraq. Avicenna J Clin Microbiol Infect, 7(1), 34-35.

IOM Iraq. (2019). *Understanding Ethnoreligious Groups in Iraq: Displacement and return*. https://publications.iom.int/books/understanding-ethnoreligious-groups-iraq-displacement-and-return-february-2019

Jäger, P., Rammelt, C., Ott, N., & Brand, A. (2019). Narrative review: the (mental) health consequences of the northern Iraq offensive of ISIS in 2014 for female Yezidis. *International Journal of Environmental Research and Public Health*, *16*(13), 2435.

Junne, F., Denkinger, J., Kizilhan, J. I., & Zipfel, S. (2019). *Aus der Gewalt des" Islamischen Staates" nach Baden-Württemberg: Evaluation des Sonderkontingents für besonders schutzbedürftige Frauen und Kinder aus dem Nordirak. Mit E-Book inside*. Juventa Verlag ein Imprint der Julius Beltz GmbH et Company KG.

Karim, H. F., & Baser, B. (2022). Collective Memory in Post-Genocide Societies: Rethinking Enduring Trauma and Resilience in Halabja. *Review of Middle East Studies*, *56*(1), 56-72.

Kim, G., Torbay, R., & Lawry, L. (2007). Basic health, women's health, and mental health among internally displaced persons in Nyala Province, South Darfur, Sudan. *American journal of public health*, *97*(2), 353-361.

Kizilhan, J. I. (2014). Religious and cultural aspects of psychotherapy in Muslim patients from tradition-oriented societies. *International Review of Psychiatry*, *26*(3), 335-343.

Kizilhan, J. I. (2018). Zur Psychologie des islamisierten Terrors. *PiD-Psychotherapie im Dialog*, *19*(02), 73-77.

Kizilhan, J. I. (2019). *Providing psychosocial care to child soldiers living in post-IS Iraq*. JSTOR.

Kizilhan, J. I. (2020). Stress on local and international psychotherapists in the crisis region of Iraq. *BMC Psychiatry*, *20*(1), 1-8.

Kizilhan, J. I., Berger, T., Sennhauser, L., & Wenzel, T. (2023). The psychological impact of genocide on the Yazidis. *Frontiers in psychology*, *14*, 1140.

Kizilhan, J. I., Friedl, N., Neumann, J., & Traub, L. (2020). Potential trauma events and the psychological consequences for Yazidi women after ISIS captivity. *BMC Psychiatry*, *20*(1), 256. https://doi.org/10.1186/s12888-020-02671-4

Kizilhan, J. I., & Noll-Hussong, M. (2017). Individual, collective, and transgenerational traumatization in the Yazidi. *BMC Medicine*, *15*(1), 198.

Kizilhan, J. I., Noll-Hussong, M., & Wenzel, T. (2021). Transgenerational transmission of trauma across three generations of Alevi Kurds. *International Journal of Environmental Research and Public Health*, *19*(1), 81.

Kizilhan, J. I., & Steger, F. (2021). The socialpsychology of Islamist terror–interdisciplinary perspectives on violence and ISIS totalitarian structures. *Global Security: Health, Science and Policy*, *6*(1), 26-37.

Kizilhan, J. I., Steger, F., & Noll-Hussong, M. (2020). Shame, dissociative seizures and their correlation among traumatised female Yazidi with experience of sexual violence. *The British Journal of Psychiatry*, *216*(3), 138-143.

Kizilhan, J. I., & Wenzel, T. (2020). Positive psychotherapy in the treatment of traumatised Yezidi survivors of sexualised violence and genocide. *International Review of Psychiatry*, *32*(7-8), 594-605.

Kornwachs, G., Hautzinger, M., & Kizilhan, J. (2024). The importance of cultural understanding and practical solutions during the handover of a psychotherapy and psychotraumatology program in Northern Iraq into local hands. *Frontiers in psychiatry*, *15*, 1434670.

Kurdistan Regional Government. (2023, 02.12.2023). Dashboard Coronavirus (Covid-19). Retrieved 01.06.24 from https://gov.krd/coronavirus-en/dashboard/

Mohammed-Marzouk, M. R. (2012). Teaching and learning in Iraq: A brief history. In *The Educational Forum* (Vol. 76, pp. 259-264). Taylor & Francis.

Neumann, J. C., Berger, T., & Kizilhan, J. I. (2021). Development of a questionnaire to measure the perceived injustice of people who have experienced violence in war and conflict areas: Perceived Injustice Questionnaire (PIQ). *International Journal of Environmental Research and Public Health*, *18*(23), 12357.

Rahman, A., & Hafeez, A. (2003). Suicidal feelings run high among mothers in refugee camps: a cross-sectional survey. *Acta Psychiatrica Scandinavica*, *108*(5), 392-393.

Shehata, D., Al-Hadeethi, B., Ibrahim, Z., Al-Lami, B., Qader, S., Maqdasy, R., Mohammad, A., Nabee, V., Saber, S., & Abdulkarim, L. (2021). The COVID-19 pandemic in the Kurdistan region of Iraq. HPHR Journal(29).

Shorsh, S. (2007). Anfal. *The Iraqi State's Genocide against the Kurds*, 1-88.

Steger, F., & Kizilhan, J. I. (2022). Usable and useful help in literature database search? A pedagogical implementation and the evaluation of an interactive screencast for Iraqi university students. *Technology, Knowledge and Learning*, *27*(3), 993-1020.

Taha, P. H., & Abdurrahman, S. M. H. (2020). Traumatic events and post-traumatic stress among Iraqi kurdish "anfal" survivors. *Duhok Medical Journal*, *14*(1), 77-91.

Taha, P. H., & Slewa-Younan, S. (2020). Measures of depression, generalized anxiety, and posttraumatic stress disorders amongst Yazidi female survivors of ISIS slavery and violence. *International Journal of Mental Health Systems*, *14*, 1-10.

Tay, A. K., Riley, A., Islam, R., Welton-Mitchell, C., Duchesne, B., Waters, V., Varner, A., Moussa, B., Alam, A. M., & Elshazly, M. (2019). The culture, mental health and psychosocial wellbeing of Rohingya refugees: a systematic review. *Epidemiology and Psychiatric Sciences*, *28*(5), 489-494.

Wolf, S., Seiffer, B., Hautzinger, M., Farhan Othman, M., & Kizilhan, J. (2019). Establishment of psychotherapeutic care in the Duhok district of North Iraq: Foundation of the Institute of Psychotherapy and Psychotraumatology and execution of a masters degree course in psychotherapy and psychotraumatology. *Psychotherapeut*, *64*, 322-328.

World Health Organization. (2020, 31.07.2020). *Rolling updates on coronavirus disease (COVID-19)*. Retrieved 01.06.24 from https://www.who.int/emergencies/diseases/novel-coronavirus-2019/events-as-they-happen

CHAPTER 8

ASSESSING THE IMPACT – OUTCOMES AND ACHIEVEMENTS OF THE IPP

JAN ILHAN KIZILHAN, JULIA BECKMANN AND ANNA WEIGELT

Since its foundation in 2016, the Institute for Psychotherapy and Psychotraumatology (IPP) worked to to enhance healthcare services in northern Iraq in the fields of education, research, prevention, and treatment (see Figure 8-1). The chapter gives a summary of the outcomes and achievements of the IPP. It covers a description of resources accumulated over the years, an evaluation of the Master of Advanced Studies of Psychotherapy and Psychotraumatology (MASPP), and the outcomes of the IPP's services, including its clinics and suicide hotline. Additionally, the chapter examines the impact of the institute's research efforts and its sustainability practices and concludes with an internal evaluation based on interviews conducted with key stakeholders, providing insights into the overall effectiveness and areas for improvement.

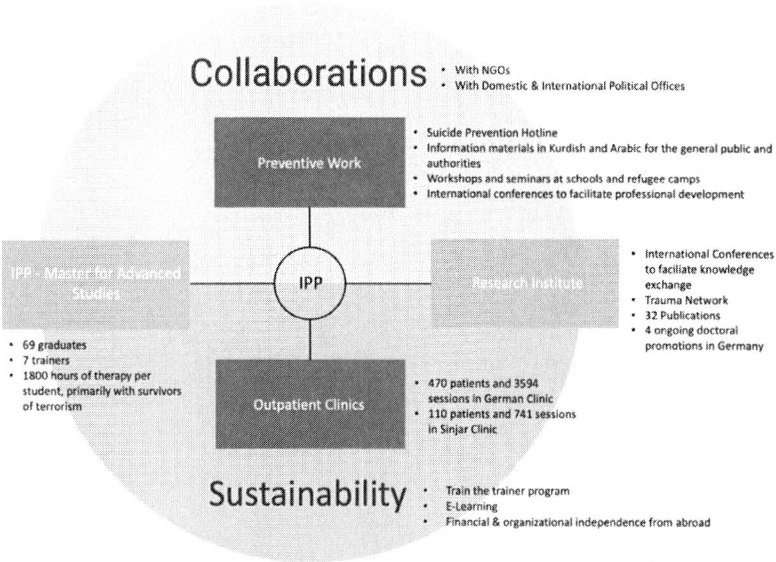

Fig. 8-1 Achievements of the IPP

IPP's Resources

The IPP is located in a university building on the campus of the University of Duhok. It includes a lecture hall, administration offices, and meeting rooms equipped with computers, printers, and other office supplies. The IPP has two administrative employees.

The IPP cooperates closely with the Duhok General Directorate of Health, Azadi Hospital, and local and international NGOs (e.g. SEED, Jiyan Foundation). A list of the IPP's cooperating partners are listed in Table 1.

Table 8-1 List of IPP's Cooperating Partners

Organization	Cooperation from	until
Duhok General Directorate of Health	2017	Ongoing
Jiyan foundation for human rights	2018	Ongoing
SEED foundation	2018	Ongoing
The Lotus Flower	2022	2022
Jesuit Refugee Services	2022	2022
Yazada	2022	2022
Suliminya Mental Health Center	2018	2020
Un Ponte Per Organization	2018	2020
Norwegian Church Aid (NCA)	2018	2020
International Medical Corps	2018	2020
Friends of Waldorf Education (FWE)	2018	2020
Springs of hope foundation	2018	2020
French Red Cross (FRC)	2018	2020
International Organization for Migration	2018	2019

Teaching at IPP

A total of 69 graduates, across three cohorts, have completed the master's program (see Table 8-2). A fourth cohort started the Master of Advanced Studies of Psychotherapy and Psychotraumatology (MASPP) in May 2023 and is expected to graduate in March 2026.

Table 8-2 Students of the IPP

Cohort	Gender		Religion			Total
	Male	Female	Muslim	Yazidi	Christian	
MASPP 17	12	16	21	5	2	28
MASPP 18	17	4	19	2	0	21
MASPP 20	10	10	14	6	0	20
MASPP 23	9	19	24	4	0	28
Total	48	49	78	17	2	**97**

Five students from the first cohort and two students from the second cohort were chosen to be trained as local lecturers in the "Train the Trainer program" (TOT). The five lecturers from the first cohort began supporting the international experts as co-lecturers in the second year of education for the second master's cohort. In the third cohort, all lectures were held by an international or local expert, together with a TOT. Three of the TOTs are pursuing their doctoral studies at the same time. Two of the TOTs are trained to conduct group self-experience sessions, where participants explore their own emotions and experiences, under the supervision of German or international psychotherapists.

On average, students completed 27 weeks of theoretical training, which comprised of 57 seminars over 117 days. Personal experience groups, supervision, intervision groups, exams, and study organization were also part of the training blocks. Training blocks usually took place four times per year. Additionally, students had to be present at the IPP for weekly or biweekly training days including intervision groups, supervision, English classes, and oral presentations. See Table 8-3 for details about theoretical training at the IPP.

Table 8-3 Theoretical Training at the IPP

Cohort	Year of master's	Weeks of training	Seminar days	Seminars
MASPP 17	1st year	8	43	17
	2nd year	13	52	21
	3rd year	9	32	12
	Total	**30**	**127**	**50**
MASPP 18	1st year	9	35	23
	2nd year	11	34	17
	3rd year	7	46	12
	Total	**27**	**115**	**52**
MASPP 20	1st year	7	34	26
	2nd year	8	39	20
	3rd year	8	37	24
	Total	**23**	**110**	**70**

A total of 61 experts from Germany, Iraq, the UK, the Netherlands, Sweden, Austria, and the USA held lectures at the IPP (39 German, 6 international, and 16 local experts). On average, 17 lecturers were needed for each study year. The number of local lecturers increased over time (see Table 8-4 for details).

Table 8-4 Lecturers at the IPP

Cohort	Year of master's	German lecturers	Other international lecturers	Iraqi lecturers	Total
MASPP 17	1st year	10	2	2	14
	2nd year	16	2	3	21
	3rd year	8	2	2	12
	Total	**21***	**3***	**6***	**30***
MASPP 18	1st year	6	1	7	14
	2nd year	10	2	3	15
	3rd year	4	2	7	13
	Total	**11***	**2***	**13***	**26***
MASPP 20	1st year	6	1	12	19
	2nd year	12	3	9	24
	3rd year	11	1	12	24
	Total	**19***	**4***	**18***	**41***

Note. Some lecturers taught seminars in several study years and are therefore counted in several years/cohorts, but the total number only counts those lecturers once.

In order to guarantee the quality of the MASPP, students regularly evaluated lectures using online surveys. The lecturers formulated study objectives for their lectures (e.g. "I can explain essential CBT approaches"). On a six-point Likert scale, the students assessed the degree to which they believed they achieved the study objectives posed by the lecturers. For the first two cohorts, more than 50% of the students agreed with the statements, confirming that they believed they reached the study goals over the course of the whole program. The percentage of students not believing that they achieved the study goals was very low (see Table 8-5).

Table 8-5 Student Perception of Achievement of Study Objectives

"I achieved the study objectives posed by the lecturers"							
Cohort	**Year of master's**	**1 (absolutely)**	**2**	**3**	**4**	**5**	**6 (not at all)**
MASP P 17	1st year	27.6%	30.2%	22.7%	13.5%	5.6%	2.2%
	2nd year	30.0%	36.5%	20.7%	10.0%	2.1%	1.2%
	3rd year	15.2%	39.8%	27.0%	11.8%	5.0%	0.3%
MASP P 18	1st year	20.8%	30.9%	24.4%	11.2%	6.1%	3.5%
	2nd year	21.3%	38.2%	17.2%	10.8%	4.5%	2.9%
	3rd year	43.0%	35.4%	14.2%	6.3%	0.9%	0.3%
MASPP 20	1st year	19.1%	38.1%	18.7%	10.2%	5.6%	1.2%
	2nd year	22.6%	29.0%	23.0%	13.7%	8.0%	1.7%
	3rd year	9.9%	29.6%	24.1%	21.1%	7.2%	3.4%

Higher percentages of students not feeling like they were able to reach the study goals in the first cohort might indicate a mismatch between the abilities of the students and requirements of the program. Adaptations of the program over time seem to have improved this in the second cohort. The MASPP 20 cohort data suggests a lower level of agreement on study objectives attainment. Contextual factors such as the global COVID-19 pandemic, international travel restrictions, staff overload, and local challenges likely impacted student evaluations. Despite these difficulties, the cohort demonstrated resilience, successfully completing their studies through a blend of in-person and online formats. The adaptability of the program in adverse conditions underscores its effectiveness and sustainability, emphasizing the need for flexible approaches in establishing psychotherapy institutes.

Evaluations of individual and group supervision demonstrate high satisfaction among the students (see Table 8-6 for student evaluations). Students felt that they had a chance to introduce their cases during the supervision, had enough time to discuss their patients, were able to improve their psychotherapeutic skills, and were able to speak openly during the supervision. They were satisfied with suggestions given by supervisors and felt that they were able to follow the proposed approaches in their work with patients.

Table 8-6 Evaluation of Supervision

"I had the chance to introduce my cases during supervision"							
Co-hort	**Year of master's**	**1 (absolute-ly)**	**2**	**3**	**4**	**5**	6 (not at all)
MASP P 17	Individual Super-vision	78.9%	5.3%	0.0%	15.8%	0.0%	0.0%
	Group Super-vision	60.0%	16.0 %	12.0 %	0.0%	8.0%	0.0%
MASP P 18	Individual Super-vision	58.8%	17.7 %	5.9%	0.0%	0.0%	5.9%
	Group Super-vision	47.1%	11.8 %	11.8 %	5.9%	5.9%	5.9%
MASP P 20	Individual Super-vision	83.3%	0.0%	5.6%	0.0%	11.1 %	0.0%
	Group Super-vision	72.2%	11.1 %	5.6%	0.0%	11.1 %	0.0%
"There was enough time to discuss my cases"							
Co-hort	**Year of master's**	**1 (absolute-ly)**	**2**	**3**	**4**	**5**	**6 (not at all)**
MASP P 17	Individual Super-vision	68.4%	10.5 %	5.3%	15.8%	0.0%	0%

	Group Super-vision	52.0%	16.0 %	16.0 %	0.0%	8.0%	0.0%
MASP P 18	Individu al Super-vision	58.8%	5.8%	5.8%	5.8%	0.0%	11.8 %
	Group Super-vision	58.8%	5.9%	11.8 %	5.9%	5.9%	0.0%
MASP P 20	Individu al Super-vision	77.8%	5.6%	0.0%	5.6%	5.6%	0.0%
	Group Super-vision	66.7%	16.7 %	0.0%	5.6%	11.1 %	0.0%
"I was able to improve my skills as a psychotherapist through supervision"							
Co-hort	**Year of master's**	**1 (absolute-ly)**	**2**	**3**	**4**	**5**	**6 (not at all)**
MASP P 17	Individu al Super-vision	57.9%	21.1 %	5.3%	10.5%	0.0%	0.0%
	Group Super-vision	52.0%	12.0 %	16.0 %	12.0%	0.0%	0.0%
MASP P 18	Individu al Super-vision	29.4%	41.2 %	0.0%	0.0%	5.9%	5.9%
	Group Super-vision	35.3%	23.5 %	11.8 %	11.76 %	5.9%	5.9%
MASP P 20	Individu al Super-vision	66.7%	16.7 %	5.6%	5.6%	5.6%	0.0%
	Group Super-vision	38.9%	33.3 %	16.7 %	5.6%	5.6%	0.0%

"I was able to speak openly during the supervision sessions"							
Co-hort	**Year of master's**	**1 (absolute-ly)**	**2**	**3**	**4**	**5**	**6 (not at all)**
MASP P 17	Individual Super-vision	68.4%	21.1 %	5.3%	10.5%	0.0%	0.0%
	Group Super-vision	48.0%	20.0 %	16.0 %	0.0%	8.0%	0.0%
MASP P 18	Individual Super-vision	64.7%	17.7 %	5.9%	0.0%	0.0%	0.0%
	Group Super-vision	47.1%	17.7 %	11.7 %	5.9%	5.9%	5.9%
MASP P 20	Individual Super-vision	61.1%	22.2 %	0.0%	11.1%	5.6%	0.0%
	Group Super-vision	50.0%	22.2 %	11.1 %	16.7%	0.0%	0.0%
"I was satisfied with the suggestions provided by the supervisor"							
Co-hort	**Year of master's**	**1 (absolute-ly)**	**2**	**3**	**4**	**5**	**6 (not at all)**
MASP P 17	Individual Super-vision	63.2%	21.1 %	5.3%	10.5%	0.0%	0.0%
	Group Super-vision	44.0%	24.0 %	16.0 %	8.0%	0.0%	0.0%
MASP P 18	Individual Super-vision	41.2%	29.4 %	0.0%	5.9%	5.9%	0.0%

	Group Super-vision	41.2%	17.7 %	17.7 %	5.9%	5.9%	0.0%
MASP P 20	Individual Super-vision	66.7%	11.1 %	16.7 %	0.0%	5.6%	0.0%
	Group Super-vision	50.0%	16.7 %	22.2 %	0.0%	11.1 %	0.0%
"I was able to follow the proposed method applied in the supervision sessions"							
Co-hort	**Year of master's**	**1 (absolute-ly)**	**2**	**3**	**4**	**5**	**6 (not at all)**
MASP P 17	Individual Super-vision	68.4%	21.1 %	0.0%	15.5%	0.0%	0.0%
	Group Super-vision	40.0%	24.0 %	20.0 %	0.0%	8.0%	0.0%
MASP P 18	Individual Super-vision	29.4%	23.5 %	11.8 %	17.7%	0.0%	0.0%
	Group Super-vision	29.4%	29.4 %	11.8 %	0.0%	5.9%	11.8 %
MASP P 20	Individual Super-vision	66.7%	16.7 %	0.0%	11.1%	5.6%	0.0%
	Group Super-vision	33.3%	44.4 %	16.7 %	0.0%	5.6%	0.0%

IPP's Services

The IPP has several cooperating partners, mainly local and international NGOs. Students of the IPP often complete their internships or practical activities in one of the NGOs, usually located in the refugee camps.

The 28 students in the first cohort treated 842 patients in 11.563 therapy sessions as part of the practical parts of their master's studies between 2017 and 2019. The 21 students in the second cohort treated 891 patients in 12.452 sessions between 2018 and 2021. The 20 students in the third cohort treated 921 patients in 14.477 sessions between 2020 and 2023. On average, each student treated 39 patients and conducted 576 treatment sessions (MASPP17: 30 patients and 413 sessions; MASPP18: 42 patients and 593 sessions; MASPP20: 46 patients and 723 sessions).

Furthermore, the German Clinic for Psychotherapy has operated since February 2021. It currently has eight psychotherapists, who are all graduates from the IPP, and one physician working there. From the time it opened, up until September 2023, 470 patients have been treated in the German Clinic for Psychotherapy. Like the German Clinic, another branch in Sinune is staffed by four psychotherapists who are dedicated to assisting individuals who suffer psychological distress as a result of displacement and war in the Sinjar region. In 2023, a total of 110 patients underwent 741 therapy sessions at the Sinjar Clinic, with an average of 7 sessions per patient.

Another service offered by the IPP is the Emergency Suicide Prevention Hotline, which is staffed by four psychotherapists. A total of 574 calls reached the hotline by September 2023. The number of calls per year has been steadily increasing from 115 calls in the first year to 217 calls in 2022, and 242 calls by September of 2023.

IPP's Research Activities

Over the past few years, the IPP has organized three international conferences. These conferences were titled the "First International Conference on Genocide and Trauma," "East meets West," and "Psychotherapy in Conflict and Post-Conflict Regions." Concurrently, collaborative efforts have resulted in the creation of 32 scientific papers. Currently, five graduates from the IPP are also pursuing doctoral studies in Germany. In partnership with the Ministry of Health in Duhok, the German Agency for International Cooperation GmbH (Deutsche Gesellschaft für Internationale Zusammenarbeit GmbH, GIZ), and several NGOs, the IPP has established a trauma network. This network is dedicated to fostering a long-term and stable network among medical, psychological, and nursing professionals, as well as academics and researchers engaged in the care of extremely traumatized individuals.

Through international conferences and scientific paper contributions, the IPP enhances Duhok's reputation as a center for cutting-edge research in trauma and conflict studies. The trauma network, on the other hand, not only boosts local expertise but also creates a sustainable infrastructure for ongoing care. This multi-faceted approach, coupled with ongoing collaboration among professionals, positions Duhok to excel in trauma care, attracting expertise and international partnerships. The IPP's efforts lay the groundwork for a resilient and self-sustaining ecosystem that will benefit the well-being of the community in northern Iraq.

Sustainability

Transition of Project Ownership

To ensure long-term sustainability, the IPP project must gradually transition from German support to local stewardship. This shift requires collaboration from key stakeholders including the University of Duhok, Ministry of Higher Education, Ministry of Health, Regional Government, political leaders, and local NGOs. The goal is for trained local lecturers to manage the project within the framework of the University of Duhok, ensuring its administration and funding.

Capacity Building and Local Leadership

Training of trainers participants initially supported external experts as co-lecturers, gradually assuming more responsibility. Today, they primarily plan, organize, and lead lectures independently, with minimal support. They have developed their own criteria for assessing student work, providing supervision, and leading sessions, with occasional input from international experts. Local lecturers now cover most topics, with intermittent input from international experts.

Challenges in Legal Recognition and Healthcare Infrastructure

Despite advancements in psychotherapy's reputation, legal recognition and frameworks are pending, leaving therapists in unclear professional conditions. Political and bureaucratic hurdles, such as the requirement for doctoral degrees to teach Master's students, also hinder local lecturers' ability to lead the project. Additionally, the absence of health insurance leads to financial challenges for the profession, highlighting the need for sustainable economic support and legal reforms. Addressing this requires advocating for policy changes.

Financial Sustainability

Although the project has received funding, the eventual end of German support will mean that sustainable financing is required from local sources. Integration into mental health and educational systems is crucial for long-term viability. Unfortunately, full financial commitment from local authorities is still pending, requiring continued advocacy efforts.

In summary, significant progress has been made in empowering local stakeholders and building capacity for project leadership. However, challenges persist in legal recognition, healthcare infrastructure, and financial sustainability. Advocacy for policy changes, increased local research opportunities, and securing full financial commitment from local authorities are essential steps to ensure the project's long-term sustainability.

Internal evaluation

The outcomes described demonstrate that the founding of the IPP, and introduction of the master's program, was a success and initiated an important process. To further evaluate the successes and challenges of the process so far, we conducted interviews with a number of project stakeholders from different areas, including: political supporters, administrative staff, lecturers, supervisors, students, TOT participants, IT staff, and administration from Germany, Iraq, and other countries. The goal was to understand the crucial steps of setting up a project like this.

Semi-structured interviews were conducted between June 2021 and April 2022. Seven interviews with German project staff were conducted in-person, four interviews with German or international interviewees were conducted online, and three interviews were written. Interviews with Iraqi interview partners were conducted in Duhok at the IPP or the German Clinic for Psychotherapy. Interviews usually lasted between 60-90 minutes. The insights from the interviews are described below.

Basic Prerequisites for the Pilot Project

For a project like the one described, the interview participants (IPs) emphasize the importance of good, long-term planning. This should involve a prior assessment of needs and of reliable structures in Germany and abroad. This includes a great wealth of experience of the project managers, as well as good project partners and reliable cooperation abroad. Planning should also consider the "unplannable." The IPs also think it is important to consider local and cultural conditions and not to "impose" anything upon them. All these basic prerequisites were considered to be present in the project.

The German and international IPs emphasized the topicality of the problem. There was consensus of a real need on the ground in the KRI due to the high number of traumatized people in combination with the lack of psychotherapeutic services available. Interviewees from the KRI emphasize the ongoing difficulties in Iraq in general, especially in the Duhok region. They also point out the challenges in the numerous camps where both Syrian refugees and internally displaced persons (IDPs) continue to be housed on a long-term basis. The project was also seen as an opportunity to be able to combat causes of flight on the ground. Through the involvement of students in the practical work, an immediate and direct effect could be achieved, despite the overall focus on long-term, sustainable change.

"... Usually there is a "memorandum of understanding" in which the goals are formulated, i.e. what you want to do, how you want to do it; the roles and the tasks within the project are also defined, so there should be no misunderstandings in this respect either..." (IP 12).

Lesson learned #1: Thorough holistic planning with needs assessment, experienced project managers, reliable partners, and adaptability for unforeseen circumstances are vital to conduct a project of this scope. Project managers should have experience and know the culture of the target country.

Teaching at the IPP

International and German IPs fulfilled most of their activities from their home countries. Lecturers and personal experience trainers flew to Duhok a few times in order to conduct seminars. Due to the COVID-19 pandemic, seminars had to be canceled and conducted online. As a result, the TOT participants took on more responsibility in supporting the international lecturers earlier than planned. The IPs rated their satisfaction with the trainers and their performance as very high. The collaboration was described as being on an equal footing, which has led to ongoing contact beyond the trainers' tasks, including joint research projects. During the pandemic, the trainers proved to be an important resource. Although they were "thrown in at the deep end," they quickly adapted to the new challenges. In retrospect, early involvement of the trainers in the lectures was useful. According to the IPs, the trainers proved to be very helpful, particularly with regard to language and cultural understanding with the students.

In carrying out the various tasks (teaching, supervision, personal experience sessions, administration, organization, technical support), the IPs emphasize the importance of good communication and a good flow of information. The collaboration between the international team was considered to be successful. Joint reflection appears to be essential, especially when working in a post-conflict region with a different culture.

"... Of course, we also understood that they were thrown in at the deep end... Now, in retrospect, I would say, yes, that was maybe a good thing... It was great to see that we had many concerns, perhaps rightly so, but that they subsided over time... It was fascinating to see what really great personalities you have there..." (IP 4)

Lesson learned #2: The early training of local lecturers is crucial, especially in terms of cultural exchange and language understanding. Utilizing local trainers and participants as resources, who can take on responsibilities and support international lecturers, is highly effective. This approach not only supports project sustainability but also fosters deeper local engagement and capacity building.

Lesson learned #3: Flexibility and quick adaptation to new challenges, such as the shift to online seminars during the COVID-19 pandemic, is also crucial for project success. Good communication and information flow are essential for successful cooperation in international teams.

Working and Conducting Therapy in the KRI

Traveling to a post-conflict region was worrying for some international staff. The IPs said that although they noticed increased security measures on site, such as armed security personnel and increased checks, they felt safe overall in Duhok. Concerns were alleviated by on-site assistance and driving services, as well as trust in the project officers and their assessment of the security situation. Interruptions due to sudden alarms were only reported once, otherwise the IPs did not notice any particular disruptions due to being in a post-conflict region.

The consequences of the conflicts could be felt in the working conditions of the therapists on-site. Many students do their practical hours in refugee camps. In some cases, the international lecturers visited these camps or had the students report on them. Problems such as lack of space, lack of privacy in therapy rooms, difficult living conditions in the camps, lack of security, as well as climate-related intense heat in the tents, have been reported as disruptive factors to conducting psychotherapy. According to local IPs, stigmatization of mental illness and high cost of transportation are other hindering factors.

Furthermore, the IPs highlight unique aspects of therapy in northern Iraq due to regional and cultural conditions. These include patients with a low level of education, culturally different views of disease models and therapy goals, or varying therapeutic attitudes. An important cultural issue for the IPs was to find a balance between imparting Western therapeutic values and core beliefs, while respecting the local culture and making possible adaptations to therapy on-site. It is considered valuable to have therapists on the ground who are well versed in the local culture. At the same time, the importance of supporting the therapists through personal experience sessions and supervision is emphasized in order to ensure good self-care. IPs express respect for the therapists' work under very difficult conditions. The application of therapeutic methods in another culture was also viewed to have great potential for informing further development of methods. There is great interest in observing these developments.

"...When it comes to the topic of psychoeducation, for example, things get interesting. How can I communicate a disorder to German patients and how can therapists in Iraq communicate a disorder to patients? The students come up with great suggestions, saying it is fine how you explain things in the West. But that's not how it is here, that's not how it works. And then there were really great discussions about how can you convey an understanding of a disease in such a way that it fits into the world of the patient?..." (IP 1)

In addition to the aforementioned cultural aspects of psychotherapy, general cultural differences were observed. The IPs reported positively on their encounters with the people in the KRI, emphasizing the hospitality and joy of getting to know each other culturally. Differences were noted in terms of intercultural cooperation. A more hierarchical way of thinking was reported, which required adjustments in the communication style. In some cases, strongly hierarchical thinking makes it difficult to trust cooperation at face value. In teaching, there is also a rather hierarchical, rigid way of thinking. Students need to be encouraged to think creatively and freely. Due to the more collective way of thinking, students find it difficult to talk about themselves and their own issues in the group. The lecturers need to adapt their approach in these circumstances as well. It is important to always reflect on communication and to work out common communication styles that work for everyone.

Lesson learned #4: Safety for the project staff in a post-conflict region must be ensured through robust on-site support and security measures.

Lesson learned #5: Working conditions in a post-conflict region can disrupt a smooth therapy process and have to be considered. Therapists might face significant challenges such as lack of privacy, difficult living conditions in refugee camps, and stigma around mental illness. Addressing hierarchical and collective cultural tendencies requires adapting communication and teaching styles to encourage more open and creative engagement from students.

Lesson learned #6: Effective therapy in post-conflict regions like the KRI requires balancing Western therapeutic values with respect for local cultural beliefs and practices.

Challenges

With regard to teaching, the IPs observed that students with bachelor's degrees generally had a lower level of academic preparation than expected. There were sometimes large differences between students in this regard. A frequently noted difficulty was that students did not always have sufficient knowledge of English, which made communication about complex issues challenging. A culturally different approach to punctuality and time arrangements was reported as a challenge by the IPs, as well as a lack of participation in online seminars. It also emerged that many students primarily used the Internet through their cell phones, which posed a particular challenge to the design of e-Learning content. Special challenges also arose from having numerous different international lecturers, such as difficulties in ensuring continuity in the delivery of e-Learning content. It also became apparent that teaching therapeutic methods which were adapted to local conditions (e.g., considering culture, post-conflict challenges, and more difficult working conditions) was not comfortable for all international experts.

Suggestions for addressing the difficulties in teaching emphasize the need for a pragmatic approach when adapting Western educational standards to the KRI. The existing bachelor's system should be taken into account, and expectations of student performance should be adjusted accordingly. According to the IPs, the selection of lecturers should not be based on internationally recognized expertise, but should also consider didactic skills and openness to adapting content to local conditions. The early use of local experts is also suggested. Regarding participation in online seminars, it is suggested that students participate in them while seated in the classroom, with the trainers present for support, to increase participation and improve comprehension. Similarly, e-Learning content should be adapted for mobile use from the outset. Another suggestion is to improve online access to technical literature and to expand the physical library.

Structural problems and suggestions for improvement focus primarily on establishing legal foundations, further developing the training concept, and ensuring the right personnel are on-site.

Lessons learned #7: Teaching methods and expectations must be adjusted to accommodate students' varying degrees of academic preparation, as well as their language proficiency. The selection of lecturers should prioritize didactic skills and adaptability to local conditions, over international recognition.

Lesson learned #8: E-Learning content should be designed for mobile accessibility from the outset, to cater to the primary mode of internet access for many students. To improve participation and comprehension in online seminars, students should attend these sessions in classrooms with local support staff present.

Future prospects

The IPs agree that good foundations have been laid through the work done so far. Apart from some smaller, concrete projects that are due in the near future (handover of technical aspects, access to literature, promotion of smooth processes), the IPs are satisfied with what has been achieved. Regarding the handover of the project to the University of Duhok, there are concerns about whether the goal of sustainability can be achieved. Interviewees from KRI express the need for continued international support. In particular, funding from the KRI is mentioned here, but there are also doubts about human resources.

Although the existing trainers are competent and motivated, there are only a few. In addition, it is important to keep the graduates motivated through appreciation, the creation of professional opportunities, and adequate pay. There is a noticeable uncertainty among the trainers as to whether, and how, the project will continue. It is necessary to create clarity, particularly through the legal anchoring of the profession and clarification of the socio-legal status of psychotherapists. There is also a desire for graduates and trainers to continue to gain clinical and scientific professional experience. This is essential for maintaining existing services and to further develop and research therapy methods in the field.

There is agreement that there is still a long way to go to achieve all these goals. Ideas have been expressed for future projects and changes that could be even further reaching. Examples include an adaptation of the bachelor system, creation of continuing education opportunities for psychotherapists, and an expansion of services for patients. An expansion of services for patients could be in the form of self-help groups or a hybrid path with MHPSS approaches, where existing psychotherapists train and supervise lay people to reach more patients. The IPs stressed the importance of cooperation with psychiatrists and religious leaders.

"... As is so often the case in the area of humanitarian aid, many things work great at the beginning as long as there is money. When you no longer have money from external sources, things no longer work. And now we have two challenges: First that the University of Duhok actually steps in and takes over financial responsibilities, and at the same time that we have enough human resources to continue..." (IP 1).

"... Now the ball is in the court of decision-makers in Duhok and in Erbil. However, we must also see that the region is still a crisis area and finance is coming from Baghdad..." (IP 10).

"... I think it's like everywhere. You have to pay them well, too. You have to create the structures so that it's also an option for them to work as a lecturer in the longer term..." (IP 3).

"... we must think beyond their time at the IPP and what they go on to do, where are they likely to work? What is the career progression for them as they get older? What would keep them in those jobs? Because that's what you want. What keeps them there? Is it going to be things around flexible working childcare? What would make it attractive to them because you must think about them as a workforce, not just as students now..." (IP 6).

"... I believe you must accompany it. And I also think you must be there. Over and over again. It's just time. It takes time. It takes time.... this next generation must grow up now..." (IP 5).

Lessons learnt #9: Achieving sustainability requires ongoing international support, especially in funding and human resources. The competence and motivation of existing trainers must be bolstered with professional opportunities, adequate compensation, and clear legal and socio-professional status. Continued development of the project includes adapting the education system, offering continuing education opportunities for psychotherapists, expanding patient services, and fostering collaborations with psychiatrists and religious leaders.

What's New?

Part of the evaluation of the pilot project was to assess the pros and cons of this new kind of academic training in comparison to the previously mentioned existing MHPSS approaches. In the discussions with the IPs, exciting perspectives emerged on the importance of the project for the future, as well as arguments and ideas for the compatibility of both approaches.

The IPs highlighted the different attitude with which students and trainers are treated in the academic setting: they are regarded as colleagues on an equal footing, not as laypeople simply carrying out something they have been taught. As mentioned earlier, scientific collaborations resulted from the work between academics and students/trainers. It was emphasized that a certain humanistic attitude was imparted through the academic training; the students not only learn about therapy, but they receive a humanistic and intellectual stimulation. Throughout their education, personal development takes place, students are empowered to think freely and creatively, and are thus able to develop confidence in their own competencies. A professional identity is formed, students come to understand basic therapeutic mechanisms and the individual, profound development that is inherent to a therapeutic process. As a result, they can make treatment decisions independently, adapt therapy methods to their patients, and develop methods further in a culturally specific way. The training therefore achieves not only better psychosocial care in the region, but also advancement on intellectual and scientific levels. Local IPs add that NGOs working under the MHPSS approach are often inadequate, and in some cases even harmful. They would often only offer relaxation exercises or briefly address trauma without sufficiently following up with the patients.

These are elements in which academic training differs from MHPSS approaches. Nevertheless, the advantages of MHPSS approaches are not to be ignored; within a short period of time, many laypersons can be trained and many patients can be cared for. Thus, the two approaches complement each other well, and MASPP graduates may be able to pass on their knowledge to laypersons.

"... these are the wonderful things that can happen about sharing ideas that make a tangible difference to people's lives, by sharing what you might be knowing with excellent clinicians working on the ground and working with them as equals, as colleagues, not as, here I am with my brilliant idea. So we tried to make it together, culturally appropriate and it was co-created with them, we didn't go, here you are, here's your menu..." (IP 6).

"... there has to be some place or there has to be some threshold where you say, ah, someone reports in with "I'm all shaken up," there has to be a diagnostic decision made somewhere by someone: 'Oh, you have OCD, it's treated that way, so go see that person.'..." (IP 2).

"... We can also convey a kind of empowerment to the therapists on site, through passage through this hard, difficult school of therapy according to Western standards. It has, I think, a high importance for the self-perception of therapists. It is also important for the therapist to have faith in his own therapy. (...) That it is not about going through a therapy manual from A to Z, but that it is about filling this theoretical knowledge with life." (IP 1).

Summary

The IPs perceived the project as an impressive, well-thought-out project that also takes cultural aspects into account. The goals set out in the project application are considered to have been achieved. Networking has also taken place locally and the project has had an influence on public perceptions. The image of psychotherapy has changed, and important local allies have been gained. Both the security situation and the pandemic were challenging, and the advantage of virtual structures became clear.

"... The project has thus done more than lay a foundation for care and therapy in a crisis area; it has also broken-down cultural skepticism about psychotherapy on the ground. The local people have recognized that altruistic help is being offered, including and especially to women and children, who are among the most vulnerable victims of war. We have also spoken with dignitaries on the ground and with the relevant ministers in order to achieve a continuation of the work on the ground..." (IP 10).

"... In projects like this, there is no such thing as failure or defeat, maybe just not the right time yet. We were also lucky. The time was right, and we just went for it..." (IP 10).

"... That's why you do it as well: I gave them something, told them something. Now they can go new ways. And maybe they're going to go and treat a Yazidi woman and it will make the difference, and that's why I'm doing it. I'm proud because I feel I use my time well to help somebody else to do something useful in the world..." (IP 6).

When asked about successes of the pilot project, the IPs praise the openness of the University of Duhok, the international collaboration, as well as the TOT program. IPs report positively on the students' high willingness to learn, and on the exchange of knowledge on a collegial level. Students and graduates of the IPP are seen as equal colleagues. It was observed that the students benefit from the MASPP and that personal development takes place in the course of their studies. The necessary adaptations in the face of the pandemic were viewed as well managed, and the use of e-Learning was described as successful. Locally, a network of collaborations with psychiatrists is emerging; jobs are available for graduates, and knowledge about psychotherapy is successfully spread via social media and word-of-mouth. It was positively noted that despite all cultural differences, psychotherapy is working across cultures and therapeutic mechanisms, with certain adaptations in methods.

"...what I think is quite great is the selection of people that is made. They are quite wonderful people. On a personal level, it's super easy to get in and work with these people. They're curious, they're joyful, ... they have an incredible willingness to learn. It's a blast to work with these people. ... I also have the feeling that the training is good for the people. So my impression is, when you see them for the first time, and then you see them again later, they are more mature..." (IP 5).

"... it's a wonderful thing, because I feel like we're directly sharing our knowledge..." (IP 6).

RESULTS FROM THE EXTERNAL EVALUATION

THOMAS WENZEL AND REEM ALKSIRI

The review process

An independent evaluation of the project was agreed upon with the Scientific Section on "Psychological Aspects of Persecution and Torture" of the World Psychiatric Association (WPA), in addition to the internal review and outcomes analyses presented in the preceding chapter. Professor Dr. med. Thomas Wenzel (TW), a Psychiatrist and licensed psychotherapist, specialist in transcultural Psychotraumatology, was asked to conduct the external project evaluation, with support from the section's Arabic-speaking legal advisor, Mag. Int. Law Reem Alksiri. This evaluation aimed at reviewing the Duhok project strategy and their implementation, following the considerations and relevant international research summarized in the earlier chapters. This review also aimed at creating a matrix that could be used in similar projects in the unfortunately growing number of war and (post) conflict settings. Some conclusions regarding the early project stages and preparation were already included in an earlier chapter of this book, and some issues in need of future project activities are described later in this chapter. It should be noted that the evaluation did not include aspects such as patient treatment outcomes nor an economic assessment or financial auditing, which are to be provided by the donors and partner Universities.

Two experienced assistant researchers, Anna Weigelt and Julia Beckmann, were recruited to support production of reports, research activities, conducting additional interviews with German project team members and stakeholders, and subsequent publications. All project reports, materials, and outcomes were provided by the team for the review. As part of the review, repeated visits were also made to the project sites, refugee camps, the psychotherapy service institution built as part of the project (German Clinic for Psychotherapy in Duhok), and to those religious institutions (especially the "Lalish" Yazidi religious institution) of special relevance to the community, the last being an ancient site not directly linked to the project. Meetings were held with key figures, including Yazidi religious leaders (like a "Pir", the important "Baba Sheik" and other leaders), NGOs, and local partner University representatives. In addition, these visits and meetings were augmented by independent qualitative interviews with randomly selected local trainees, members of the local team, as well as a group of experts trained in the project or otherwise benefitting from it, materials and documentation reviewed separately by the project team and international experts.

A written agreement, funding, and a memorandum of understanding (MOU) was drawn up to aid the process, with the budget for the evaluation provided by the main donor (German Ministry of the Exterior). When the project evaluation was instigated, a checklist (attached as part of this book and filled out for the project) and a publication were already under preparation. They were developed by the involved WPA section members to be shared with WPA and can be expected to promote the criteria for mental health care in war and conflict areas, but were already used for the project and consequent evaluation. The checklist integrated experiences from multiple projects, experts, and MHPSS concepts. It was added to the list of internal review, feedback, and quality management (QM) structures. The evaluation also served to appraise and improve the checklist and guidelines.

Joint publications and future activities for sustainable long-term development were agreed upon with the team leaders. These activities include addressing long-term concerns like protection of culture, victim reintegration, online services, forensic trainings, psychotherapy legislation development, and advanced science teaching. To protect the independence of the external evaluation, the external reviewers were not involved in the teaching or local project implementation during the time span of review process, but participated in publication of joint results.

The evaluation was accompanied by research, such as collecting and analyzing relevant articles from medical and other fields. This was shared with the team as part of the feedback process. A triangulation method was used to create a thorough review of the different evaluation criteria. This method incorporated both internal and independent external sources as outlined above. The review included the already mentioned WPA section checklist, a comparison of the original project aims (taken from the project documents), interviews conducted by the external reviewers, and outcome materials from the project record collection. The evaluation (review) is designed as a report, but also as part of this book, to share information on integrated health care models and resources developed to support other projects in similar settings. It will be followed by a second book summarizing the results of the general research described above and the project with a second large international publisher as secondary project outcome with concrete recommendations for the roles of different stakeholders. Further publications have summarized specific project results and have been published in international scientific journals, or submitted to journals at the time when this chapter was written. A selection of the most relevant outcomes, such as the Perceived Injustice Questionnaire (PIQ), developed in the project, and information materials used in the community, are parts of this book's attachments.

General results

The evaluation process came to the following conclusions:

A) Aims fulfilled:

1) The explicitly stated a-priority primary aim of the project was to provide the base for culturally-sensitive, sustainable, low-barrier psychotherapy services, facilitated by the key objective of offering a long-term professional psychotherapy education embedded in a major regional University and integrated with regional health care challenges and special needs, especially in the field of Psychotraumatology.
2) This primary aim was later extended to reflect the additional needs and opportunities identified during the project. Specifically, the building of capacity in international scientific research and expansion of the network of the local partner university became additional priorities. This would benefit all prospective patients and stakeholders, including religious community leaders, local and international NGOs, international universities, and organizations such as the UN bodies, the WPA, and European governments and foundations. These entities can provide support to continue the project in future, augmenting the limited local resources. Both the primary and additional aims were fulfilled to a high degree. The team established a strong and potentially sustainable core institution and local team to provide professional psychotherapy. The team also collaborated effectively with local and international stakeholders. This included the internationally supervised University-based training structure, practice opportunities in the German Psychotherapy Clinic, and collaborations with NGO services. These additions helped address the previously limited availability of free or low-cost public health services.

B) Means and methods used in the project

Means and methods used in the project can be seen as adequate, professional, and economical, especially considering the difficult pre- and post-crisis conditions, such as high levels of psychological trauma, the lack of legal process to provide justice and security, and numerous barriers present against the provision of services. That barriers include limited local transport facilities, stigma against mental health, stigma against survivors, traditional culture, and continuous insecurity and danger. The project takes all factors, including culture, into account and we view it as a model that can be adapted for similar cultures, settings, and situations.

C) Future perspectives and considerations

Future approaches could include more art and media-based therapies, especially for children. An extension of online services could also be useful, along with additional trainings in specific subjects. These subjects could include forensic examinations of human rights violations and domestic violence, as well as research strategies like qualitative methods and MHPSS approaches.

Most of these potential future activities could also be offered to other members of faculties in the University, NGOs, and external health care and social services. Due to ongoing problems in the region, continued international support for the project is recommended for a limited time to ensure long-term sustainability, supplementing the measures already taken. This may lead to a larger group of trained psychotherapy professionals, the development of new services, better acceptance and decreased stigma, further improvement of professional standards, and stronger embedding of the local University and healthcare structures within international scientific and professional networks. Regarding the last aspect, further close collaboration with international Universities and professional umbrella organizations like the World Psychiatric Association and the European Association for Psychotherapy was initiated during the evaluation phase of the project and will be part of long-term activities.

Vulnerable groups and groups with further needs identified during the project, steps taken and future needs in their support

Women

As previously noted, women were a prime target of the terrorist ISIS/DAESH group (Jager et al., 2019). They were exposed to abduction, sexual violence, and slavery, leading to severe long-term psychological trauma symptoms. Before the project, there were numerous significant challenges in this regard in the communities. Access to health care was limited, and perpetrators often acted with impunity. There was mistrust of neighbors, who may have been complicit in abductions by creating lists of women available for abduction[1]. Additionally, there were substantial barriers to their reintegration and acceptance in a traditionally reclusive and religiously influenced community upon their return. Issues around reintegration were exacerbated when women were married to, and especially had children with, the non-Yazidi perpetrators (Kizilhan, 2020).

One of the first steps taken by the project team leaders was to immediately evacuate groups of Yazidi women to Germany, with the support of the German Government (the "Special Quota project"). This provided them with a protective environment within a strong Yazidi exile community and access to treatment for trauma. This effort was part of a unique worldwide humanitarian admission program (HAP) (Hillebrecht, 2018) and was later repeated for selected groups of women with special needs. Rometsch et al. (2018, 2020), also conducted research on this groups. The authors reported that "the predominant psychological symptoms the care providers noticed were fear, depressive symptoms, feelings of guilt, and sleep and eating disorders. Regarding somatic symptoms, the care providers mainly received complaints about pain in the head, back, chest, and stomach. Helpful strategies for providing adequate health care were care providers' cooperating with physicians, precise documentation of beneficiaries' symptoms, and additional support in directing the beneficiaries through the health care system" (Rometsch (2020). This confirmed the need for professional psychotherapy especially for this group.

Several steps were taken to give special attention to women during the project. These included providing outreach services to camps and engaging with religious community leaders to generate community support for

[1] Interview with a survivor and team members by TW

the re-acceptance of women who had been abducted and were now still living in refugee camps as local displaced persons (DPs) due to the previously mentioned barriers. A female gatekeeper/receptionist was employed in the German Clinic for Psychotherapy, to reduce barriers in help-seeking and bridge traditional stigmas. Female students have also been enrolled in the psychotherapy training program. Still, women require continuous attention in these situations due to the described challenges.

Children

In all conflict regions, children are a major group of victims, even if not directly exposed to atrocities. In Iraq, several subgroups with special needs should be considered. Child soldiers need a comprehensive placement and rehabilitation program[2], as has been shown in other regions. Children conceived from women abducted by ISIS will not be accepted by their mother's communities and might not be recognized as members of the Yazidi religion. This further aggravates the mothers' situation (Kizilhan, 2019, 2020), in addition to the trauma and conflicts caused by the rape that resulted in these births. Psychological health of children was part of the training curricula but might require further efforts.

The elderly and communities

The elderly can be especially vulnerable, considering the long-term impact of transgenerational trauma and the frequently observed increase in PTSD symptoms in this group (Six-Hohenbalken, 2019). At the same time, they could also be important leaders and advisors in their communities. They should be supported in these leadership roles, if possible, but the concept has not been sufficiently researched and would require more consideration.

Persons at risk for suicide

Earlier research has observed an increase in suicidal ideation in situations like those in Iraq (Wenzel, 2009). This may reflect a feeling of hopelessness and might not be the same as a concrete suicide risk. However, it remains an important issue and was addressed by a special project

[2] See https://www.hrw.org/news/2016/12/22/iraq-armed-groups-using-child-soldiers-0

("Emergency Suicide Prevention Hotline") within the general activities of the newly established institutions in Iraq.

References

Hillebrecht J, Helmes A, Bengel J. [Psychological Care for a High-Risk Group of Refugees - Concept of Care for the Yazidi Women and Children of the Sonderkontingent Baden-Wurttemberg in Freiburg]. Psychother Psychosom Med Psychol. 2018;68(3-4):137-41.

Jager P, Rammelt C, Ott N, Brand A. Narrative Review: The (Mental) Health Consequences of the Northern Iraq Offensive of ISIS in 2014 for Female Yazidis. Int J Environ Res Public Health. 2019;16(13).

Kizilhan JI. Changes in the Yazidi Society and Religion after the Genocide—A Growing Rapprochement with Human Rights? Open Journal of Social Sciences. 2019;7:7-17.

Kizilhan JI, Friedl N, Neumann J, Traub L. Potential trauma events and the psychological consequences for Yazidi women after ISIS captivity. BMC Psychiatry. 2020;20(1):256.

Kizilhan JI, Steger F, Noll-Hussong M. Shame, dissociative seizures and their correlation among traumatised female Yazidi with experience of sexual violence. Br J Psychiatry. 2020;216(3):138-43.

Rometsch-Ogioun El Sount C, Denkinger J K, Windthorst P, Nikendei C, Kindermann D, Renner V, et al. Psychological Burden in Female, Iraqi Refugees Who Suffered Extreme Violence by the "Islamic State": The Perspective of Care Providers. Front Psychiatry. 2018;9:562.

Rometsch C, Denkinger JK, Engelhardt M, Windthorst P, Graf J, Nikendei C, et al. Care providers' views on burden of psychosomatic symptoms of IS-traumatized female refugees participating in a Humanitarian Admission Program in Germany: A qualitative analysis. PLoS One. 2020;15(10):e0239969.

Six-Hohenbalken M. May I be a sacrifice for my grandchildren-transgenerational transmission and women's narratives of the Yazidi ferman. Dialect Anthropol. 2019;43(2):161-83.

Wenzel, T., et al. Suicidal ideation, post-traumatic stress and suicide statistics in Kosovo. An analysis five years after the war. Suicidal ideation in Kosovo. Torture 2009; 19(3): 238-247.

APPENDICES

Appendix A: Perceived Injustice Questionnaire (PIQ)

Perceived Injustice Questionnaire for survivors of mass violence and atrocities in war and conflict areas.

Please choose for each statement to what extent you agree with it.	**Strongly agree**	**Agree**	**Neither agree nor disagree**	**Disagree**	**Strongly disagree**
A1 It is worth fighting for justice.	☒	☒	☒	☒	☒
EEC5 I feel a lot of anger, rage or aggression.	☒	☒	☒	☒	☒
RF4 I cannot forgive the people who did not help me.	☒	☒	☒	☒	☒
IE3 Some of the experiences that I have had were a lot worse than what humans generally experience.	☒	☒	☒	☒	☒
A3 People need to hear my story.	☒	☒	☒	☒	☒

RF3 I do not want to forgive, I want revenge.	☒	☒	☒	☒	☒
Please choose for each statement to what extent you agree with it.	**Strongly agree**	**Agree**	**Neither agree nor disagree**	**Disagree**	**Strongly disagree**
A5 I am hopeful that the people, who are responsible for the acts of injustice, will be legally held accountable.	☒	☒	☒	☒	☒
EEC6 I feel guilty and/or ashamed.	☒	☒	☒	☒	☒
IP3 I often get less than I deserve.	☒	☒	☒	☒	☒
EEC7 I feel humiliated.	☒	☒	☒	☒	☒
IP4 I am suffering because of someone else's negligence.	☒	☒	☒	☒	☒
IP5 It all seems so unfair.	☒	☒	☒	☒	☒
EEC2 I feel unsafe.	☒	☒	☒	☒	☒
IE2 I feel that acts of injustice that I have experienced affected me in a permanent way.	☒	☒	☒	☒	☒
EEC1 I am scared that I will experience injustice again in my life.	☒	☒	☒	☒	☒

Please choose for each statement to what extent you agree with it.	**Strongly agree**	**Agree**	**Neither agree nor disagree**	**Disagree**	**Strongly disagree**
IP2 My life is a lot harder than the lives of people around me.	☒	☒	☒	☒	☒
IE1 Some of the experiences that I have made were wrong and acts of injustice.	☒	☒	☒	☒	☒
RF1 Nothing will ever make up for what I have gone through.	☒	☒	☒	☒	☒
A2 If another person treats me in an unjust or wrong way, I can successfully protest against it.	☒	☒	☒	☒	☒
IP1 I am mistreated more often than other people.	☒	☒	☒	☒	☒
EEC3 I feel betrayed by humanity and cannot trust many people.	☒	☒	☒	☒	☒
A4 Other people's compassion helps me when dealing with injustice.	☒	☒	☒	☒	☒
EEC4 I feel left alone.	☒	☒	☒	☒	☒
RF2 I want to punish the person who has hurt me.	☒	☒	☒	☒	☒

Appendix B: Publications published as project results

Beckmann J, Wenzel T, Hautzinger M, Kizilhan JI. (2022). Training of psychotherapists in post-conflict regions: A Community case study in the Kurdistan Region of Iraq. Front Psychiatry. 2022 Aug 22;13:947903. doi: 10.3389/fpsyt.2022.947903. PMID: 36072460; PMCID: PMC9442973.

Denkinger, J., Windthorst, P. El Sount, C., Kizilhan J.I., Zipfel, S., Junne, F. (2018). Secondary traumatization in caregivers working with women and children who suffered extreme violence by the 'Islamic State, Frontiers, 5:9:234 Psychiatry doi: 10.3389/fpsyt.2018.00234

Gerdau, I., Kizilhan, J.I., Noll-Hussong, M. (2017). PTSD and related disorders among female Yazidi refugees following ISIS attacks. Frontiers; doi.org/10.3389/fpsyt.2017.00282 IF 3.161

Jan Ilhan Kizilhan & Thomas Wenzel (2020) Positive psychotherapy in the treatment of traumatised Yezidi survivors of sexualised violence and genocide, International Review of Psychiatry, DOI: 10.1080/09540261.2020.1809356

K. Adorjan, S. Mulugeta, M. Odenwald, D. M. Ndetei, A.H. Osman, M. Hautzinger, S. Wolf, M. Othman, J. I. Kizilhan, O. Pogarell, T. G. Schulze (2017). Psychiatrische Versorgung von Flüchtlingen in Afrika und dem Nahen Osten - Herausforderungen und Lösungsansätze. Nervenarzt, DOI 10.1007/s00115-017-0365-4.

Kizilhan J, Wenzel T (2020) Concepts of Transgenerational and Genocidal Trauma and the Survivors of ISIS Terror in Yazidi Communities and Treatment Possibilities. Int J Ment Health Psychiatry 6:1. doi: 10.37532/ijmhp.2020.6(1).174

Kizilhan JI (2020) Impact of Sexual Violation of ISIS Terror against Yazidi Women after Five Years. JSM Sexual Med 4(1): 1025. IF 3.65

Kizilhan JI and Neumann J (2020) The Significance of Justice in the Psychotherapeutic Treatment of Traumatized People After War and Crises. Front. Psychiatry 11:540. doi: 10.3389/fpsyt.2020.00540

Kizilhan JI, Berger T, Sennhauser L and Wenzel T (2023) The psychological impact of genocide on the Yazidis. *Front. Psychol.* 14:1074283. doi: 10.3389/fpsyg.2023.1074283

Kizilhan, J., Salman, R. (2015). Die Psychologie des islamischen Terrors. Trauma und Gewalt, 9; 4, 328-342.

Kizilhan, J.I (2019). Providing Psychosocial Care to Child Soldiers Living in Post-IS Iraq, ICCT Research paper May 2019, DOI: 10.19165/2019.1.05 ISSN: 2468-0486

Kizilhan, J.I. (2016). Vergewaltigung als Waffe. Loyal, Zeitschrift für Sicherheitspolitik, 6/2016, 26-31.

Kizilhan, J.I. (2018). Posttraumatic stress disorder among former ISIS child soldiers in northern Iraq, British Journal of Psychiatry (BJP). doi.org/10.1192/bjp.2018.88 IF

Kizilhan, J.I. (2018). PTSD of Rape after ISIS ("Islamic State") captivity. Archive of Women Health, https://doi.org/10.1007/s00737-018-0824-3

Kizilhan, J.I. (2018). PTSD, Pain Medication and Addiction of refugees in Iraq. Trauma Stress Disorder and Treatment, 7:2 DOI: 10.4172/2324-8947.1000186

Kizilhan, J.I. (2018). Transkulturelle Aspekte bei der Behandlung der Posttraumatischen Belastungsstörung. Zeitschrift Trauma und Gewalt.DOI 10.21706/TG-12-3-0

Kizilhan, J.I. (2018). Zur Psychologie des islamisierten Terrors. Psychotherapie im Dialog (PiD), 19:73-77

Kizilhan, J.I. (2019). Changes in the Yazidi Society and Religion after the Genocide—A Growing Rapprochement with Human Rights? Open Journal of Social Sciences, 2019, 7, 7-17,

Kizilhan, J.I. (2019). Mental Health on Collective Trauma and Terror on Yazidi in Iraq. World Journal of Advance Health Care Reserarch, 3,(6):122-128

Kizilhan, J.I. (2020). Stress on local and international psychotherapists in the crisis region of Iraq. *BMC Psychiatry* 20, 110 (2020). https://doi.org/10.1186/s12888-020-02508-0

Kizilhan, J.I., Cavelius, A. (2017). Traumata. In den Händen des IS. Gehirn und Geist, 7 (2017): 32-40.

Kizilhan, J.I., Friedl, N., Neumann, J. Traub, T. (2020). Potential trauma events and the psychological consequences for Yazidi women after ISIS captivity. *BMC Psychiatry* 20, 256 (2020). https://doi.org/10.1186/s12888-020-02671-4 IF 3.3

Kizilhan, J.I., Neumann, J. (2020). The Psychological Impact of Terrorism in North Iraq: Study of Posttraumatic Stress Disorder and Associated Factors in Victims of 2007 Bombings in Northern Iraq. International Journal of Women Health, accepted IF 2.0

Kizilhan, J.I., Noll-Hussong, M. (2017). Individual, Collective and Transgenerational Traumatization in the Yazidi, BMC Medicine 2017, 15:198, doi.org/10.1186/s12916-017-0965-7

Kizilhan, J.I., Noll-Hussong, M. (2020). The psychological impact of COVID-19 in a refugee camp in Iraq. Psychiatry and Clinical Neurociences. DOI:10.1111/pcn.13142.

Kizilhan, J.I., Noll-Hussong, M., Wenzel, T. (2021). Transgenerational Transmission of Trauma across Three Generations of Alevi Kurds. *Int. J. Environ. Res. Public Health,* 19(1):81, DOI:10.3390/ijerph19010081

Kizilhan, J.I., Steger, F. (2021) The socialpsychology of Islamist terror – interdisciplinary perspectives on violence and ISIS totalitarian structures, Global Security: Health, Science and Policy, 6:1, 26-37, DOI: 10.1080/23779497.2021.1927796

Kizilhan, J.I., Steger, F., Noll-Hussong, M. (2020). Shame and dissociative seizures and their correlation among traumatized female Yazidi with experience of sexual violation. BJP. 216, 138–143. doi: 10.1192/bjp.2020.2

Mirzaei S, Kizilhan JI, Alksiri R, Wenzel T (2022) Women as Human Rights Defenders at Risk - A Present Case Example. ARCH Women Health Care Volume 5(1): 1-2.

Neumann JC, Berger T, Kizilhan JI. (2021). Development of a Questionnaire to Measure the Perceived Injustice of People Who Have Experienced Violence in War and Conflict Areas: Perceived Injustice Questionnaire (PIQ). Int J Environ Res Public Health, 24;18(23):12357. doi: 10.3390/ijerph182312357. PMID: 34886079; PMCID: PMC8657181.

Steger, F., Kizilhan, J.I. (2021). Usable and Useful Help in Literature Database Search? A Pedagogical Implementation and the Evaluation of an Interactive Screencast for Iraqi University Students, Technology, Knowledge and Learning, https://doi.org/10.1007/s10758-021-09523-4

Wolf, S., Seiffer, B., Hautzinger, M., Othman M.F., Kizilhan, J.I. (2019). Aufbau psychotherapeutischer Versorgung in der Region Duhok, Nordirak. Gründung des Instituts für Psychotraumatologie und Psychotherapie sowie Durchführung eines Masterstudiengangs für Psychotherapie und Psychotraumatologie. Psychotherapeut 2019 · 64:322–328, https://doi.org/10.1007/s00278-019-0344-2

Appendix C: Suicide Prevention Brochure

our hotline number:

80025050

IF YOU ARE SOMEONE WHO IS THINKING ABOUT SUICIDE:

1. Wait, do not undertake any action to hurt yourself.
   You do not have to act on your suicide thoughts.
   Your thoughts and attitudes can be changed.
2. Before taking any action talk to someone,
   it could be a family member or a close friend.
3. Call this hotline to support you.
4. If it is difficult for you to call, send us a message please.
5. Try to keep yourself safe for now and move to another place.
6. Try to realize that this is a temporally situation.
   Keep in mind there are other reasons to live.

committing suicide is not the right solution for your current problems.
Your critical situation is temporary. We understand your dilemma
but be sure we have better solutions for you.

CALLING OUR HOTLINE NUMBER IS FREE

WARNING SIGNS

THAT FAMILY AND FRIENDS SHOULD KNOW

If one of your relatives or a friend has the following signs or if you notice that his/her thoughts or behaviors are changing and has negative thoughts regarding life.
YOU CAN CONTACT US
to save one's life from death.

TALKING ABOUT:

* Wanting to die.
* Being a burden to others.

FEELING:

* Hopeless, traped, or having no reason to live.
* Extremely sad, more anxious, agitated or full of rage.
* Great guilt or shame.
* Unbearable emotional or physical pain.

CHANGING BEHAVIORS SUCH AS:

* Planing or searching ways to commit suicide.
* Withdrawing from friends, saying goodbye and writing a will.
* Display extreme mood swings.
* Taking dangerious risks such as driving extremely fast.
* Eating or sleeping more or less.
* Using drugs or alcohol more often.

If these warning signs apply to you or someone you know get help as soon as possible specially if the behavior is new or has increased recently.

Appendix D: German Clinic Brochure

Clinic Work Modality

- The clinic will help you to overcome your personal problems through listening, talking, and practical exercises.
- The clinic helps clients to boost their confidence and calmness.
- The staff of clinic are trained in scientific methods to relieve clients distress.
- The therapist helps the clients to find better solutions for problems.
- All information are kept confidential.

IPP German Clinic for Psychotherapy

Free of charge

A healthy mind creates a healthy body

ippgcp.org

info@ippgcp.org

ippgerman_clinic_psychotherapy

Gali Road - College of Health Sciences

SCAN ME

0751 549 66 17

Working days from **Sunday** to **Thursday**

Working Hours **02:00** pm to **07:00** pm

About

The IPP German clinic for psychotherapy was founded in 2021 by the institute of psychotherapy and psychotruamtology /University of Duhok in cooperation with the German universities in the state of Baden Wurttemberg. The core funder of the clinic is the German government as well as the university of Duhok. Services in the clinic are free for all papulations.

After our country went through many types of massacres, genocides and traumas, still continuing until now, many people started to feel unhappy or sad in their everyday lives, and to have excessive thoughts about what happened. This Clinic is a place where people can express themselves, process the difficulties in their lives, and get help in professional, scientifically tested ways.

The Clinic Consists of

- The Medical Part: it consists of one general physician who will check the psychical health and exclude medical issues.
- The Psychiatric Part: The psychiatrist will assess and manage the therapeutic in the clinic.
- Psychotherapy Part: The professional psychotherapists hold master degree and well trained in the field of the psychotherapy. The therapy is through talking and using professional techniques to resolve psychological issues.

Clinic Services

Who should visit the Clinic? You can visit the Clinic ...

- If something bad happened to you and you can't handle it alone and you feel uncomfortable.
- If an accident happened to you and the memories of that trauma bother you.
- If you faced a problem either inside the family or outside of it that makes you anxious and you don't know how what to do or decide.
- If your sleep and/or appetite are changed and you are not like before.
- If you lost a loved one and can't adjust yourself with this loss.
- If you have such fear of some thing or place that your normal life is badly affected.
- If you have certain behaviors or thoughts which are not normal to you and you can't control or stop them.

There are many more difficulties which can cause distress; the staff of clinic will support and help you with them.

Appendix E: Sinjar Clinic Brochure

Clinic Work Modality

- The clinic will help you to overcome your personal problems through listening, talking, and practical exercises.
- The clinic helps clients to boost their confidence and calmness.
- The staff of clinic are trained in scientific methods to relieve clients distress.
- The therapist helps the clients to find better solutions for problems.
- All information are kept confidential.

ippgcp.org
sinjarclinic@ippgcp.org
Duhok, Kabarto 1 Camp-DOLSA Center

SCAN ME

0751 200 25 21

IPP Sinjar Clinic for Psychotherapy

Free of charge

Your mental health is just as important as your physical health!

Working days from Sunday to Thursday

Working Hours 09:00 am to 02:00 pm

About

The IPP Sinjar clinic for psychotherapy in Kabarto 1 camp was founded in 2022 by the institute of psychotherapy and psychotruamtology /University of Duhok in cooperation with the German universities in the state of Baden Wurttemberg. The core funder of the clinic is the German government as well as the university of Duhok. Services in the clinic are free for all populations.

After our country went through many types of massacres, genocides and traumas, still continuing until now, many people started to feel unhappy or sad in their everyday lives, and to have excessive thoughts about what happened. This Clinic is a place where people can express themselves, process the difficulties in their lives, and get help in professional, scientifically tested ways.

The Clinic Consists of

- The Medical Part: it consists of one general physician who will check the psychical health and exclude medical issues.
- The Psychiatric Part: The psychiatrist will assess and manage the therapeutic in the clinic.
- Psychotherapy Part: The professional psychotherapists hold master degree and well trained in the field of the psychotherapy. The therapy is through talking and using professional techniques to resolve psychological issues.
- The social Work Part: the clinic has two social workers in the camp, who approach people and promote clinic activities and services.

Clinic Services

Who should visit the Clinic? You can visit the Clinic ...

- If something bad happened to you and you can't handle it alone and you feel uncomfortable.
- If an accident happened to you and the memories of that trauma bother you.
- If you faced a problem either inside the family or outside of it that makes you anxious and you don't know how what to do or decide.
- If your sleep and/or appetite are changed and you are not like before.
- If you lost a loved one and can't adjust yourself with this loss.
- If you have such fear of some thing or place that your normal life is badly affected.
- If you have certain behaviors or thoughts which are not normal to you and you can't control or stop them.

There are many more difficulties which can cause distress; the staff of clinic will support and help you with them.

Appendix F: Project Management Checklist

	Before	During	At project conclusion	Example	Comment
Consultation with stakeholders					
With local government					
With local health institutions					
With victims and prospective patients					
With trauma survivors					
With local health care experts					
With local academic educators					
With local religious leaders					
Analyses of local health care legislation					
Analyses of local health care infrastructure					
Identification of existing services and their needs					
Identification and MOU with local personal resources					
Identification of cultural resources					
Assessment of possible coordination with local healers					
Coordination with IASC or its components					
Coordination with UN and/or WHO agencies					
Coordination with national/local ministry of health					
Analysis of professional formation guidelines, titles, and certificates					
Identification, training, and supervision of local staff					
Identification, training, and supervision of international staff					

<table>
<tr><td>Installation of complaint and QM procedure</td><td></td><td></td><td></td><td></td><td></td></tr>
<tr><td></td><td>Before</td><td>During</td><td>At project conclusion</td><td>Example</td><td>Comment</td></tr>
<tr><td>Mechanism for feedback, review, and implementation of improvements</td><td></td><td></td><td></td><td></td><td></td></tr>
<tr><td>Identification of useful materials</td><td></td><td></td><td></td><td></td><td></td></tr>
<tr><td>Adaptation and translation of useful materials</td><td></td><td></td><td></td><td></td><td></td></tr>
<tr><td>Building a local or online library of resources for staff and trainees</td><td></td><td></td><td></td><td></td><td></td></tr>
<tr><td>International conferences and symposia for staff, community experts, and trainees</td><td></td><td></td><td></td><td></td><td></td></tr>
<tr><td>Building further international networks for the local team</td><td></td><td></td><td></td><td></td><td></td></tr>
<tr><td>Supervision or intervision for the international team</td><td></td><td></td><td></td><td></td><td></td></tr>
<tr><td>Supervision or intervision for the local team</td><td></td><td></td><td></td><td></td><td></td></tr>
<tr><td>Analysis of cultural factors including health belief models</td><td></td><td></td><td></td><td></td><td></td></tr>
<tr><td>Science teaching</td><td></td><td></td><td></td><td></td><td></td></tr>
<tr><td>Science teaching projects for trainees</td><td></td><td></td><td></td><td></td><td></td></tr>
<tr><td>Joint publications between the international and local teams</td><td></td><td></td><td></td><td></td><td></td></tr>
<tr><td>Identification of possible gender issues</td><td></td><td></td><td></td><td></td><td></td></tr>
<tr><td>Clarification of ownership</td><td></td><td></td><td></td><td></td><td></td></tr>
<tr><td>Identification, adaptation, and translation of evaluation and research tools</td><td></td><td></td><td></td><td></td><td></td></tr>
<tr><td>Development of questionnaires and review tools for issues which have not been covered</td><td></td><td></td><td></td><td></td><td></td></tr>
<tr><td>Analysis of online infrastructure and their acceptance</td><td></td><td></td><td></td><td></td><td></td></tr>
</table>

Identification and collection of local health belief models and idioms of distress					
Updates and continuous monitoring of developments by team					
Training provided as planned					
	Before	**During**	**At project conclusion**	**Example**	**Comment**
Supervision provided					
External evaluation provided					
Interim Reports provided and reviewed by donor/stakeholder					
Summary report prepared and provided					
Selected results published					
Integration with MHPSS based models					
Collaboration with legal organizations for provision of interdisciplinary collaboration					
Provision of practice for local trainees					
Anti-Stigma measures implemented					
A gender strategy developed and implemented					
A hotline established focusing on relevant issues like suicide					
An anti-suicide program established					
A plan for hand-over developed in collaboration with local stakeholders and donors					

Appendix G: Project Participants

Prof. Dr. Dr. Jan Ilhan Kizilhan	Dean
Dr. Bohar Sulaiman Issa	Vice-dean
Dr. Mamo Farhan Othman	Vice-dean
Ibrahim Khalil Musa	Admin manager
Adhm Ismael	Admin manager
Ranya Dayan Jaafer	Secretary
Hewan Omar	Secretary
Amad Ayad Mohammed	Finance Auditor
Manuela Strobel	Finance and Admin
Prof. Dr. Martin Hautzinger	Teaching Staff
Dr. Sebastian Wolf	Teaching Staff
Tersa Porsild Gali	Teaching Staff
Dr. Gabriel Kornwachs	Teaching Staff
Christiana Nolte	Teaching Staff
Florian Steger	Teaching Staff
Dr.Ines Riessen	Teaching Staff
Florian Brunke	Teaching Staff
Dr.Elisabeth Kaiser	Teaching Staff
Fischer, Melanie S.	Teaching Staff
Svaldi, Jennifer	Teaching Staff
Brankemeier, Eva-Lotta	Teaching Staff
Akbar, Sameena Mariam	Teaching Staff
Dr. Nezar Emsat Tayib	Teaching Staff
Dr. Qasim Haso Abdullah	Teaching Staff
Dr. Yousif Ali Yassen	Teaching Staff
Dr. Parjan Taha Hashim	Teaching Staff
Dr. Warjeen Sulieman Yaseen	Teaching Staff
Asmaa Ibrahim M. Salih	Teaching Staff
Mayan Ismael Hussein	Teaching Staff
Musaab Abdulhafidh Zina, IPP	Teaching Staff

Shaima Mohammed Namiq	Teaching Staff
Ibrahim Hama Saeed	Teaching Staff
Madih Hama Salih M. Amen	Teaching Staff
Kovan Ahmed Abdullah	Teaching Staff
Pershang Omar Ahmed	Teaching Staff
Dr. Ahmad Abdulbaghi	Teaching Staff
Ismail Khuadaida Adham	Teaching Staff
Dr. Assad Adnan	Teaching Staff
Prof. Dr. Qanta Ahmed	Teaching Staff
Dr. Adham Ismail Khudaida Alhaji	Teaching Staff
Prof. Dr. Ameen Hussein Asma	Teaching Staff
Ali Ismail Azad	Teaching Staff
Beather Barahmand	Teaching Staff
Dr. Katharina Bitzker	Teaching Staff
Abdalla Fatah Brwa	Teaching Staff
Prof. Dr. Hanna Christiansen	Teaching Staff
Emily Nguyen Collett	Teaching Staff
Dr. Anselm Crombach	Teaching Staff
Dr. Selin Demir	Teaching Staff
Dr. med. Katharina Dönneweg	Teaching Staff
Prof. Dr. Thomas Ehring	Teaching Staff
Prof. Dr. Thomas Elbert	Teaching Staff
Dr. Jakob Fink-Lamotte	Teaching Staff
Dr. Nadine Friedel	Teaching Staff
Rzgar M. Frmsek	Teaching Staff
Jafaar Muhammed Galavej	Teaching Staff
Dr. Uwe Artur Harlacher	Teaching Staff
Linda Hennrich	Teaching Staff

Prof. Dr. Jürgen Hoyer	Teaching Staff
Prof. Dr. Husso Khasum	Teaching Staff
Dr. Barany Lazgin	Teaching Staff
Jule Lehr	Teaching Staff
Prof. Dr. Petra Theresia Morscheuser	Teaching Staff
Musaab Arezi	Teaching Staff
Musaab Abdulhafidh Zinal	Teaching Staff
Dr. Sami Ahmed Nawzad	Teaching Staff
Johanna Neumann	Teaching Staff
Prof. Dr. Hans Reinecker	Teaching Staff
Dr. Maggie Schauer-Elbert	Teaching Staff
Dr. Laura Seebauer	Teaching Staff
Prof. Dr. Ulrich Stangier	Teaching Staff
Prof. Dr. Marina Taloyan	Teaching Staff
Alissa Ulrich	Teaching Staff
Prof. Dr. med. Barbara Wild	Teaching Staff
Dr. Sarah Wilker	Teaching Staff
Dr. Haval Y. Yacoob	Teaching Staff
Dr. Ali Youssif	Teaching Staff
Mr. Akram	Teaching Staff
Prof. Ahmed Alya	Teaching Staff
Musa Hami Hamid	Teaching Staff
Mamand Ja'afer Hastin	Teaching Staff
Hunar Assaf	Teaching Staff
Hussein Qasim Khalid	Teaching Staff
Saeed Ahmed Naeima	Teaching Staff
Khasan Hassan Nizer	Teaching Staff
Ali Hassan Saefullah	Teaching Staff